Features and Management of Acute and Chronic Neuro-Covid

Marco Cascella • Elvio De Blasio

Features and Management of Acute and Chronic Neuro-Covid

Springer

Marco Cascella
IRCCS, Fondazione G. Pascale
Istituto Nazionale Tumori
NAPOLI, Napoli
Italy

Elvio De Blasio
Emergency Unit
Multidisciplinary Emergency Unit for
COVID-19 Campania
Napoli, Italy

ISBN 978-3-030-86704-1 ISBN 978-3-030-86705-8 (eBook)
https://doi.org/10.1007/978-3-030-86705-8

This Springer imprint is published by the registered company Springer Nature Switzerland AG
The registered company address is: Gewerbestrasse 11, 6330 Cham, Switzerland

Dedicated to all colleagues and friends who are engaged at the forefront of this long-standing battle against an invisible but terrifying enemy

Foreword

At the beginning of the pandemic, in the middle of the night, I received a message from Marco asking for my opinion on a clinical case of COVID-19. He was excited because the patient's conditions rapidly improved after he received one dose of tocilizumab. As an immunologist, I understood that the pathophysiology of the disease was largely attributable to the cytokine storm and this evidence could be exploited for therapeutic purposes. In other words, what we learned over the years in immuno-oncology could be translated to the treatment of COVID-19, particularly the host inflammatory response phase of the disease. In this critical situation, it was evident that not only the lung, but all the organs were affected by the hyperinflammation with subsequent damage. In this context, the acute and long-lasting neurological manifestations of COVID-19 configure a chapter of paramount importance.

The authors have comprehensively addressed all the problems related to neuro-COVID, from the neuropathogenesis of SARS-CoV-2 infection, to the acute clinical pictures, and diagnostic approaches, to the post-acute neurological, psychiatric, and neurocognitive issue. The result is a book that is enjoyable to read and full of information. I appreciated, for example, the authors' choice to summarize the therapeutic suggestions into highlights. This strategy facilitates rapid consultation by those who may have difficulty navigating into the plethora of scientific literature on the subject and search for rapid practical suggestions. The efforts of the authors will certainly be rewarded, and I am sure that both experienced readers and those who intend to deepen their knowledge in the field will appreciate this book.

Paolo A. Ascierto
Unit of Melanoma, Cancer Immunotherapy
and Development Therapeutics
Istituto Nazionale Tumori IRCCS Fondazione G. Pascale
Naples
Italy

Preface

Similar to other epidemic-induced coronaviruses, the SARS-CoV-2 seems to be neuroinvasive, neurotropic, and neurovirulent. A Chinese study published in the first weeks after the onset of the pandemic reported neurological symptoms were present in 36% of COVID-19 patients. Subsequently, thanks to the growing number of data reported in the literature, clinicians and researchers deduced that the neurological manifestations could represent a separate chapter of the disease. The term "neuro-COVID" was coined. Nevertheless, further data must be produced to characterize its profile and obtain a precise taxonomy. In the meantime, we realize that neuro-COVID is an umbrella that collects disparate clinical manifestations. In this set, neurological effects, psychological/psychiatric aspects, and neurocognitive phenomena are included. The pathophysiology of these processes is very complex. Besides a potential direct viral damage, other mechanisms, such as immune-mediated reactions, hypoxia, effects of multiorgan dysfunction, could be involved. Furthermore, the consequences of long-term intensive care treatment, such as psychological sequelae derived from isolation in critically ill patients, should not be underestimated. These arguments also concern non-hospitalized patients who have been subjected to a high burden of psychological distress.

In neuro-COVID, a logical distinction concerns the acute forms from those that occur at a distance (Fig. 1). Although for narrative aims this approach is valid, it has many limitations. Most of the clinical pictures recognize pathophysiology that determines a trigger in the acute phase and that can clinically manifest itself within the acute manifestations of the disease, or at a distance. Therefore, there is an overlapping and difficulties in temporally placing most phenomena often arise. For example, changes in taste and smell, pain, headache, and dizziness may begin when COVID-19 explodes and persist as respiratory symptoms resolve. Nevertheless, the same clinical manifestations can occur after a free interval. Since several diagnostic and therapeutic aspects must necessarily be kept separate, in this book the distinction between acute and chronic forms is maintained.

Another issue concerns the correlation between the clinical expressions of neuro-COVID and the features of the underlying pathology. Myalgia, joint pain, sore throat, abdominal pain, chest pain, and headache usually accompany respiratory symptoms but they can also occur as isolated clinical findings, or can be expressed regardless of the severity of COVID-19. Research on pathophysiology will clarify this and other doubts. The angiotensin-converting enzyme 2/renin–angiotensin system pathway and the direct virus-induced damage, the exuberant immune-mediated inflammation, and disease-related factors represent a thriving field of research that borders on the fields of neurology and embraces multiple disciplines.

The diagnostic phase plays a very important role. Given that the different expressions of neuro-COVID can have a deleterious impact on the patient's prognosis, a high index of clinical suspicion for neurological complications is mandatory. Thus, every effort should be done to reach a definitive diagnosis. In this contest, besides a complete clinical evaluation, it is often necessary to utilize a battery of neuroimaging, laboratory, and electrodiagnostic tests. Nevertheless, organizing diagnostic pathways can be very difficult. For example, in the case of in-hospital patients, some diagnostic procedures, such as neuroimaging techniques or electrophysiological tests, could be a challenge due to the increased risk of virus transmission to other patients and staff.

A chapter of enormous interest in COVID-19 concerns the post-acute effects of the disease. The implications, in fact, are manifold and range from the need to accurately and urgently characterize the spectrum of clinical conditions that are involved, to the healthcare needs, and obviously to the health costs associated with them. An amount of scientific evidence is showing that COVID-19 is not only a pathology that affects the physical health of those who contracted it, but it can induce a series of non-negligible psychological consequences. Some symptoms related to the contracted infection such as fatigue, weakness, and pain rarely disappear immediately once the critical phase of the disease is overcome but also occur in the periods following COVID-19, impacting the quality of life of patients who have contracted the SARS-CoV-2 infection. In particular, symptoms such as fear, mood changes, states of anxiety, depression, sleep disorders, and insomnia can occur alone or in combination by structuring a variety of psychological syndromes. In the context of long-COVID, risk factors should be carefully addressed. It seems, for instance, that middle-aged women are more prone to develop debilitating long-term symptoms.

The therapy of many clinical forms of neuro-COVID is often addressed by the individual specialist according to the type of symptom, or clinical manifestation,

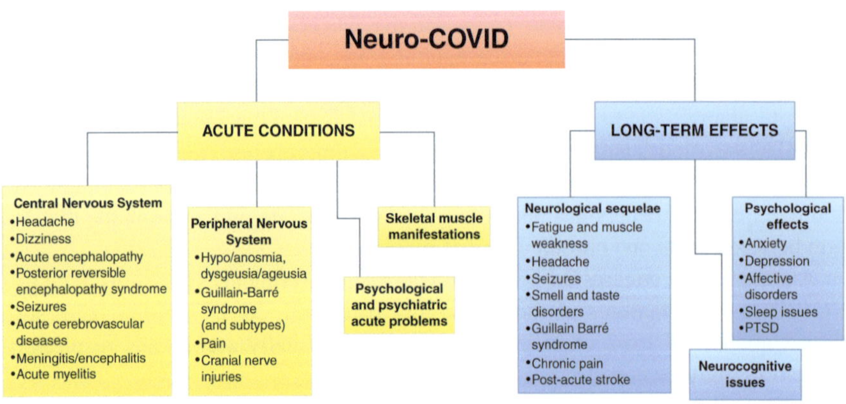

Fig. 1 Neuro-COVID: Synopsis

who follows the rules of good clinical practice. Very often, however, this approach is not enough and a multidisciplinary, or preferably interdisciplinary, strategy is desirable. It is a further challenge that launches the disease. It seems appropriate to create synergies between medical and non-medical branches that are apparently distant and to intensify efforts in the field of translational medicine.

Since research on SARS-CoV-2 and COVID-19 is advancing at unprecedented speed, much data reported in this book on the pathophysiology, clinic, diagnosis, and therapy will soon become obsolete. However, another lesson this pandemic has taught us is to speed up the timing of science disclosure. It provides the implementation of translational research and building of research programs starting from synthetic, but exhaustive, pathways, on specific topics. It is the real purpose of this manuscript. To write it, we raced against time for providing an agile and useful book to be consulted by clinicians, researchers, and even non-expert readers.

Napoli, Italy Marco Cascella
Napoli, Italy Elvio De Blasio

Acknowledgments

The list of people we should thank is particularly long. They are all those doctors, nurses, health workers who, since the beginning of the pandemic, have thrown all of themselves into the arena fighting against this indomitable beast. This book is dedicated to all of them, and from them, we have obtained a wealth of data, suggestions, most of which are not collected in scientific publications, but are an integral part of a wealth of experience that will remain indelible. This wonderful inspiration enhanced our determination and creativity.

We are especially grateful to colleagues who materially assisted us in drafting the text, especially when we faced topics that went beyond our areas of competence. In particular, we have to extend our heartfelt thanks to two doctors and researchers of the San Pio Hospital (Benevento, Italy). Dr. Marco Sparaco, a neurologist from the Division of Neurology and Stroke Unit performed an excellent revision of the chapter on clinical features of neuro-COVID. Moreover, Dr. Carmine Franco Muccio, neuroradiologist from the Division of Neuroradiology of the same hospital has offered an invaluable contribution in drafting the chapter on diagnostics.

We thank Dr. Andrea Ridolfi, Editor Clinical Medicine Books, Responsible Editor, Intensive Care Medicine, Anesthesiology, Neurology at Springer for his kind and professional coordination. The experience accumulated in the field of scientific publications allows us to affirm that his competence is far above the average. He provided us with valuable advice at each stage of our project development. These requirements are what an author expects when the best publisher to entrust his/her manuscript is sought.

Finally, special thanks go to Laura and Vincenzo Cascella, medical students. They have critically read the text and provided us with important suggestions to make it accessible not only to expert readers, but also to those who are confronted with these issues for the first time.

Contents

Abbreviations

^{18}F-FDG	^{18}F-fluorodeoxyglucose
ACE	Angiotensin-converting enzyme
ADC	Apparent diffusion coefficient
ADEM	Acute disseminated encephalomyelitis
AHLE	Acute hemorrhagic leukoencephalomyelitis
AIDP	Acute inflammatory demyelinating polyradiculoneuropathy
AMAN	Acute motor axonal neuropathy
AMSAN	Acute motor and sensory axonal neuropathy
ANE	Acute necrotizing encephalitis
Ang	Angiotensin
ANM	Acute necrotizing myelitis
ARDS	Acute respiratory distress syndrome
ASL	Arterial spin labelling
AT	Ang type
BBB	Blood-–brain barrier
BBE	Bickerstaff brainstem encephalitis
BCSFB	Blood–cerebrospinal fluid barrier
BDNF	Brain-derived neurotropic factor
BFP	Bilateral facial palsy with paresthesia
BMS	Brain midline shift
CAM	Confusion assessment method
CAR-T	Chimeric antigen receptor T
CBF	Cerebral blood flow
CBV	Cerebral blood volume
CendR	C-end rule
CNS	Central nervous system
COVID-19	Coronavirus-induced disease 2019
CRP	C-reactive protein
CRS	Cytokine release syndrome
CSF	Cerebrospinal fluid
CT	Computed tomography
CTA	CT-Angiography
CTP	CT perfusion
DCE	Dynamic contrast enhancement

DPP4	Dipeptidylpeptidase 4
DRG	Dorsal root ganglia
DSC	Dynamic susceptibility contrast
DWI	Diffusion weighted imaging
EEG	Electroencephalography
EMG	Electromyography
FLAIR	Fluid-attenuated inversion recovery
GBS	Guillain-Barré syndrome
GCS	Glasgow Coma Score
GFAp	Glial fibrillary acidic protein
GM-CSF	Granulocyte-macrophage colony-stimulating factor
HCoV	Human coronavirus
HEV	Hemagglutinating encephalomyelitis virus
HIV	Human immunodeficiency virus
ICH	Intracerebral hemorrhage
ICP	Intracranial pressure
ICU	Intensive care unit
IFN	Interferon
IL	Interleukin
IP10	Interferon gamma inducible protein-10
IVIG	Intravenous IG
MCP1	Monocyte chemoattractant protein 1
MERS	Middle East respiratory syndrome
MFS	Miller Fisher Syndrome
MHV	Murine hepatitis virus
MIP1A	Macrophage inflammatory protein 1A
MIS-C	Multisystem inflammatory syndrome in children
MMP	Matrix metalloproteinase
MRI	Magnetic resonance imaging
mRS	Modified Rankin scale
nEVs	Neuronal-enriched extracellular vesicles
NICE	National Institute for Health and Care Excellence
NIHSS	National Institutes of Health Stroke Scale
NIRS	Near-infrared spectroscopy
NK	Natural killer
NRP	Neuropilin
OB	Olfactory bulb
ORN	Olfactory receptor neuron
PAG	Periaqueductal gray
PD	Parkinson's disease
PET	Positron emission tomography
PICS	Post-intensive care syndrome
PNC	Polyneuritis cranialis
PNS	Peripheral nervous system
PP2A	Protein phosphatase 2A

PRES	Posterior reversible encephalopathy syndrome
PTSD	Post-traumatic stress disorder
RAS	Renin–angiotensin system
ROS	Reactive oxygen species
RT-PCR	Reverse transcriptase-polymerase chain reaction
SAH	Subarachnoid hemorrhage
SARS	Severe acute respiratory syndrome
SARS-CoV-2	Severe acute respiratory syndrome coronavirus 2
SSE	Shannon's spectral entropy
STIR	Short tau inversion recovery
SWI	Susceptibility weighted imaging
TCCD	Transcranial color-coded duplex
TCD	Transcranial cerebral Doppler
TF	Tissue factor
TLR	Toll-like receptors
TMPRSS	Transmembrane serine protease
TNF-α	Tumor necrosis factor α
US	United States
WBC	White blood cell count

Pathophysiology of COVID-19-Associated Neurotoxicity

1

1.1 Introduction

The clinical spectrum of COVID-19 (coronavirus induced disease 2019), the pandemic caused by the severe acute respiratory syndrome coronavirus 2 (SARS-CoV-2), varies from paucisymptomatic forms to clinical conditions ranging from different degrees of respiratory insufficiency to multiorgan/systemic manifestations such as sepsis, septic shock, until multiorgan failure.

Similar to SARS-CoV which is another member of the family *Coronaviridae* and responsible for the severe acute respiratory syndrome (SARS) outbreak, from 2002 to 2003, SARS-CoV-2 can spread through active pharyngeal viral shedding. In turn, extrapulmonary manifestations of COVID-19 are encompassed among the clinical features of the disease. Nevertheless, a key aspect of the COVID-19 pathophysiology is understanding whether this extrapulmonary involvement is produced by damage from viral spreading (direct damage). Moreover, it should be advisable to distinguish alterations produced by an aberrant inflammatory response to the viral attack (indirect damage) from organ damage that is the expression of advanced disease with multiorgan dysfunction or failure. The latter picture has complex pathophysiology including invasive therapies, drugs, severe hypoxia, and other causes.

Regardless of the precise underlying pathogenic mechanisms, it is remarkable that in COVID-19 several extrapulmonary manifestations frequently occur [1]. Evidence suggests that hematologic [2], cardiovascular [3], renal [4], gastrointestinal, hepatobiliary, and pancreatic [5] systems, and other organs [6–8] can be affected by the disease.

Within the context of the COVID-19-related extrapulmonary manifestations, the neurologic aspects of the disease represent a special chapter [9, 10]. The term "neuro-COVID" is useful for encompassing these neurological manifestations. Notably, neurological issues were also described in other coronavirus-induced diseases including the SARS and the Middle East respiratory syndrome (MERS), in

M. Cascella, E. De Blasio, *Features and Management of Acute and Chronic Neuro-Covid*, https://doi.org/10.1007/978-3-030-86705-8_1

2012 [11]. It was demonstrated, for instance, that SARS-CoV can provoke a wide range of lesions to the neurons, such as demyelination, and glial cells, mostly expressed as glial hyperplasia; these lesions were localized in several brain areas [12]. Previously, in 1993, and thus before the emergence of SARS and MERS, some authors conducted in vitro and in vivo experiments for evaluating the neurotoxicity of the human coronavirus HCV-229E on oligodendrocytes [13]. Later, it was also proved that primary cultures of human neural cells, adult astrocytes, and adult microglia can be infected by coronaviruses [14]. Interestingly, the awareness that many coronaviruses, not just human coronaviruses (HCoVs), can infect the central nervous system (CNS) of animals has long been known. In 1962, Greig et al. [15] isolated the hemagglutinating encephalomyelitis virus (HEV), which is a β-coronavirus, in the brains of pigs. Furthermore, in the early 1980s, two different coronaviruses were detected in autopsy neural tissues of two patients suffering from multiple sclerosis. The viruses, generically indicated with the initials of the patients and not further characterized, were also isolated in their cerebrospinal fluid (CSF) [16].

Thus, similar to other epidemic-induced coronaviruses, the SARS-CoV-2 seems to be neuroinvasive, neurotropic, and neurovirulent. Nevertheless, given the magnitude of the COVID-19 pandemic, these phenomena can have considerable importance.

Despite the great interest of the scientific community in the neuropathogenesis of SARS-CoV-2 infection, there are many open questions. The potential route of entry of the virus to the nervous tissue, the ability to damage cells, and the induction of immune-mediated processes are all issues that must necessarily be well elucidated. As mentioned above, the question is whether the clinical manifestations of neuro-COVID are the effect of direct viral damage or they are caused by an excessive immune-mediated response of the host. Is it possible an association between both mechanics? Similarly, it would be appropriate to distinguish between events that characterize acute damage to central and peripheral nervous tissue from processes that could clinically manifest at a distance. The pathophysiology of the latter could be very complex to explain. In addition to direct viral damage, other mechanisms such as immune-mediated reactions, hypoxia, effects of multiorgan dysfunction, could be involved. Furthermore, the consequences of long-term intensive care treatment, such as psychological sequelae derived from isolation in critically ill patients, should not be underestimated.

On these premises, a worrying scenario is opened and further research is needed to better clarify if the neurotoxicity can induce long-term sequelae probably manifested in terms of post-infectious neurodegenerative and neuroinflammatory complications. Previous studies, indeed, suggested that coronaviruses can provoke processes of demyelination, neurodegeneration, and cellular senescence. These changes could also accelerate brain aging and/or exacerbate neurodegenerative conditions [17].

Starting from experimental elements that come from different branches such as molecular biology, virology, neurophysiology, the study of pathophysiology must be able to arrive at an overall vision, as it happens for the construction of a mosaic. Although we are a long way from this goal, the road seems to have been drawn.

Moreover, the vast spectrum of neurological manifestations involves two types of problems. The former concerns the need for clinical care of patients who can be extremely complex to treat. On the other hand, the latter issue concerns the need to strengthen the preclinical research aimed at identifying the pathogenic mechanisms underlying the pulmonary and extrapulmonary involvement of the disease for offering clinicians better therapeutic choices [18–21].

This chapter is aimed at dissecting the pathologic mechanisms of COVID-19-associated neurotoxicity. The issue of pain mechanisms (COVID-pain) is discussed and updates on preclinical findings, ongoing clinical investigations, as well as perspectives for conducting preclinical and clinical investigations are also proposed.

1.2 Overview on Neurological Manifestations

The neuro-COVID chapter encompasses clinical manifestations of varying severity, incidence, and significance. They can manifest before fever and respiratory symptoms, or be the unique clinical manifestation of COVID-19. Additionally, clinical manifestations may also occur after the resolution of the acute phase (long-COVID). Although in most cases there are isolated neurological symptoms (e.g., headache, dizziness), complex scenarios can occur. Therefore, the term neuro-COVID is an oversimplification as it appears to be a great umbrella that collects disparate clinical conditions.

According to the location of symptoms, neurologic manifestations of COVID-19 can be grouped into three categories including central nervous system (CNS) manifestations, peripheral nervous system (PNS) manifestations, and skeletal/muscular clinical expressions. Furthermore, the onset time of the clinical presentations can help differentiate infective (acute) from post-infective complications. A classification based on the pathophysiology of the symptoms seems to be more appropriate. It should differentiate clinical conditions produced by direct damage from others related to indirect injury (e.g., neuroinflammation and cytokine-related injury), or disease-related (e.g., ischemic, multiorgan impairment) damage. Nevertheless, it is often difficult to separate the mechanisms and overlap phenomena exist.

Headache is one of the most common signs of COVID-19 (often associated with fever). It usually has a non-specific meaning. Clinically it is manifested as tension-type or migraine without aura, migraine-like headache (less commonly), with long-lasting duration and analgesic resistance. Dizziness is frequently combined with headache (and tinnitus), and is often observed in the earlier disease.

Data from literature and clinical experience suggest that olfactory and gustatory dysfunction is considered an early manifestation of COVID-19 infection [1].

Besides taste and smell disorders, which are reported by up a quarter of COVID-19 patients [22], myalgia and fatigue are common clinical manifestations. A meta-analysis found that the prevalence of myalgia is 35.8% [23], but some authors reported percentages up to 50% [24]. In another analysis ($n = 8697$), it was calculated that fatigue affects 35% of patients [25].

Neurological complications can also be serious. Of note, there are reports of stroke, encephalopathies such as steroid-responsive encephalopathy, posterior reversible encephalopathy syndrome (PRES), encephalitis, and acute hemorrhagic necrotizing encephalopathy [26]. Furthermore, a number of central, peripheral, and neuromuscular manifestations including ophthalmoparesis, facial paresis, Guillain-Barré syndrome, and its rare form Miller Fisher Syndrome, as well as symmetrical neuropathy, critical illness myopathy and neuropathy, myositis, and rhabdomyolysis have also been described [22–30].

Clinical and diagnostic aspects of neurological, psychological/psychiatric, and neurocognitive manifestations of neuro-COVID are discussed in other sections of the book. In this chapter, the issues of physiopathology will be more properly addressed.

1.3 Pathophysiology of COVID-19-Associated Neurotoxicity

Although in this area the research has produced important results, and many acquisitions have been imported according to translational research processes from other fields, multiple dark sides exist. Based on the evidence gathered so far, the neuropathogenesis of SARS-CoV-2 infection encompasses several large groups of mechanisms:

- Primary neurotropism.
- Immune-mediated and neuroinflammatory processes.
- Gut–brain axis involvement.
- Effects of multiorgan dysfunction.

Despite the SARS-CoV-2 neuroinvasion and neurotropism are debated, this approach can be useful for differentiating mechanisms and clinical forms. For instance, olfactory and/or taste disorders seem to be the effect of a direct neural injury and this, at least in part, explains why they are often recognized as early manifestations of the infection. On the contrary, acute cerebrovascular diseases can be interpreted as hypercoagulability, high systemic inflammatory response, vascular endothelial injury, and alteration of cerebral autoregulation.

Nevertheless, since overlapping between mechanisms is often inevitable, this distinction seems useful more for research purposes than for establishing a precise taxonomy of the neuro-COVID. Finally, it must be emphasized that this approach is most useful for narrative purposes (Fig. 1.1).

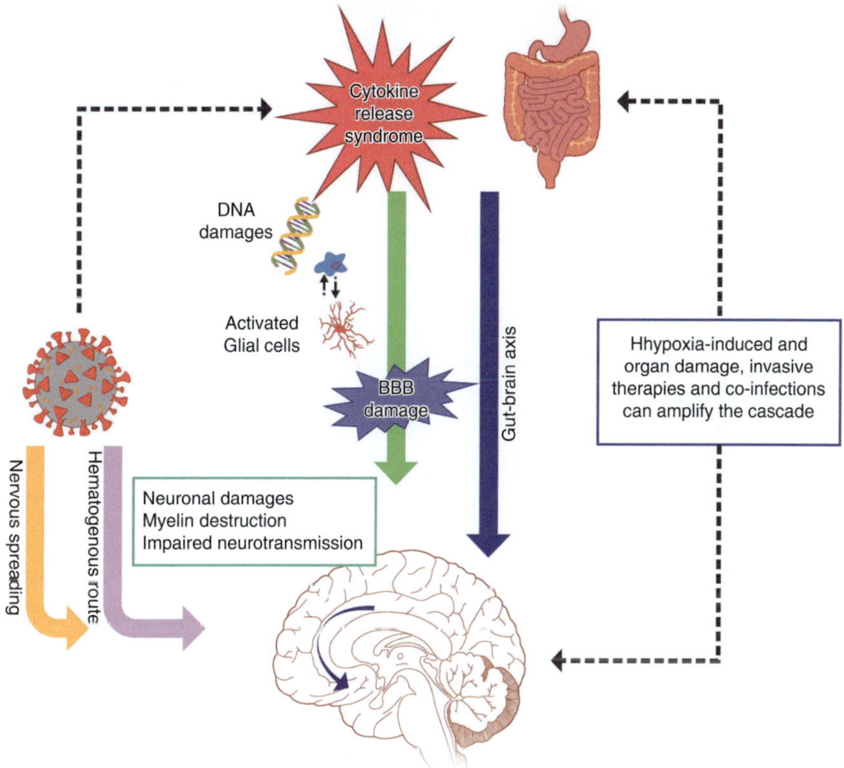

Fig. 1.1 Overview of mechanisms underlying the neuropathogenesis of SARS-CoV-2 infection. Primary neurotropism presupposes SARS-CoV-2 entry into the nervous tissue through the neurogenic or hematogenous pathway. Immune mediated and neuroinflammatory processes are mediated by the release of cytokines that induce microglial activation and damage to the blood–brain barrier (BBB) with functional and structural alterations in different brain areas. The deregulated inflammatory response can induce endothelial alterations and hypercoagulability. Gut–brain axis involvement predicts a cross-talk between the intestine and the brain through a privileged neurogenic pathway. Finally, multiorgan dysfunction with hypoxia, co-infections, and therapies can amplify the cascade or produce damage regardless of direct or indirect neurotropism

1.3.1 The Issue of SARS-CoV-2 Neurotropism

Since in microbiology organotropism is the tendency of some microorganisms to predominantly localize in certain organs or systems, neurotropism is the ability of the virus to infect human neurons and, in turn, to productively replicate within the nervous tissue.

The issue of neurotropism can be addressed by referring to two different pathogenic steps:

- The ligand (virus)–receptor (host) interaction.
- The mechanisms of diffusion towards the CNS.

The matter of the virus–receptor interaction is the basis of the virulence mechanism of each virus. In its general meaning, it concerns the ability of the pathogen to interact with the cells of the parasitized organism. As extensively demonstrated and discussed below, SARS-CoV-2 recognizes precise cell receptors. The phenomenon of organotropism, therefore, should correspond to the different expression of these receptors in different organs and tissues. This scheme appears overly simplistic, as a multitude of factors can influence this special type of bond. In addition, factors that act downstream of the receptor binding affect the efficiency of the binding itself.

The exceptional contagiousness and virulence of SARS-CoV-2 are not necessarily synonymous with extrapulmonary organotropism. Even if the receptor is almost unique for various organs and tissues, its expression and particular factors related to the tissue, largely condition virulence. In other words, in the pathogenetic chain of the infection, the virus can find peculiar or privileged tropism mechanisms in certain cells or tissues. Conversely, even if those cells and tissues express the receptor for the virus, many factors such as access to the receptor itself, and defense mechanisms, alter the effectiveness of the binding. All these conditions could characterize the issue of SARS-CoV-2 neurotropism.

Thus, key elements useful for analyzing the pathophysiology of the potential direct neurotoxicity are the general scheme of cell/tissue tropism and, consequently, the mechanisms of virulence. Although further research is needed for understanding the precise mechanisms, paramount aspects of the biological behavior of the virus have been elucidated.

From the beginning of the COVID crisis, numerous studies focused on the pathogenic mechanisms of the virus. Some important information emerged from previous research on SARS-CoV. Compared to other known HCoVs such as HCoV-OC43 and HCoV-229E that can cause common colds—these viruses cause approximately 15–30% of cases of the common cold—and self-limiting upper respiratory infections (in immunocompetent individuals), the virus responsible for the SARS marked a turning point: the evolutionary process had allowed a member of the family to gain important characteristics of virulence [31]. On the other hand, despite the genetic sequence of SARS-CoV and SARS-CoV-2 is similar for about 80%, the two viruses have important structural differences in their surface proteins and, in turn, in their viral load kinetic. Thus, both deleterious HCoVs have pathogenic characteristics that can predispose to both pulmonary and extrapulmonary organotropism.

1.3.1.1 The Evidence for SARS-CoV-2 in Nerve Tissue

Autopsy studies demonstrated a broad organotropism of SARS-CoV-2. In addition to being identified in the lungs, heart, liver, kidneys, the virus was also recognized in the brain tissues. It must be emphasized, however, that in these studies, the viral genome was identified in a minority of autopsies (8/22) and, above all, when found, the genetic material (SARS-CoV-2 RNA copies per cells) was quantitatively little relevant [32]. In other postmortem examinations of patients with COVID-19, no signs of encephalitis or CNS vasculitis were shown [33]. Overall, evidence of direct viral neurotoxicity is inconclusive and comes from small sample sizes or biased studies. For example, postmortem examinations were conducted on brains from individuals who died due to severe forms of the disease. In these settings, pathological alterations in various organs and tissues, including nervous tissue are prone to develop independently of SARS-CoV-2 infection. Moreover, similar results were described by Matschke et al. [34] who conducted autopsy tests on a considerable sample ($n = 43$).

Since autopsy studies are not conclusive, it is necessary to seek certainties in other fields of study. Interesting investigations on the subject were conducted in vitro. In a 3D human brain organoids model (pluripotent stem cells, iPSCs) previously used for studying neurological disorders [35], Ramani et al. [36] demonstrated that SARS-CoV-2 may target neurons, producing a variety of cellular alterations (e.g., Tau hyperphosphorylation) until death. Furthermore, they found that in this model SARS-CoV-2 does not effectively replicate. The authors concluded that, although SARS-CoV-2 can produce neuronal damages, the CNS may not support its active replication.

Certainty of a direct viral invasion would be obtained from the in vivo identification of SARS-CoV 2. This would mean isolating the virus in the CSF. Whatever pathway the virus has traveled including the blood torrent transport, nervous spreading, or other routes, the passage in the CSF would imply the blood–brain barrier (BBB) crossing. However, there is only scarce evidence based on isolated case reports. For example, in a 24-year-old man with meningitis/encephalitis (convulsion accompanied by unconsciousness associated with SARS-CoV-2) Moriguchi et al. [37] isolated the viral genome (reverse transcription-polymerase chain reaction, RT-PCR test) in the CSF. Furthermore, the presence of an antibody movement in CSF is not necessarily synonymous with viral invasion in this territory. In a small-size study conducted in COVID-19 patients with clinical manifestations of encephalopathy ($n = 8$), Alexopoulos et al. [38] found anti-SARS-CoV-2 antibodies (also from intrathecal IgG synthesis) in the CSF but not the viral genome, in all the subjects studied [38]. Therefore, detection of antibodies from CSF appears to be mainly indicative of extensive damage to the BBB.

Other data can be obtained from imaging investigations. In a retrospective analysis in severe COVID-19 patients ($n = 37$) with neurologic manifestations (mostly alteration of consciousness and agitation), several neuroradiologic patterns (excluding ischemic infarcts) of parenchymal injury were detected. In particular, the authors illustrated eight distinctive magnetic resonance imaging (MRI) patterns. The most frequent MRI findings were signal abnormalities located in the medial temporal lobe, non-confluent multifocal white matter hyperintense lesions on fluid-attenuated inversion recovery (FLAIR) sequence, diffusion with variable enhancement, associated with hemorrhagic lesions, and extensive and isolated white matter microhemorrhages. Of note, only one patient was positive for SARS-CoV-2 RNA in the CSF [39]. Furthermore, in a prospective study, Lu et al. [40] found that microstructural alterations in the brain parenchyma can occur during the recovery phase from COVID-19. Although all these findings are not suggestive for a direct neurotropism, they offer important data on disease-related nervous tissue damage and, most importantly, they show that the onset of CNS damage can be asynchronous with respiratory manifestations of COVID-19. The results need to be examined carefully, because of the correlation between imaging data and the potential development of long-term complications of the disease.

Taken together, these data contrast with what was previously found about SARS-CoV, in both preclinical and clinical investigations. About the pathogen responsible for SARS, more scientific evidence is available. In a transgenic mouse model for the human angiotensin-converting enzyme 2 (ACE2), Netland et al. [41] demonstrated that the entry of the virus through the olfactory pathway could produce a rapid viral spreading to the nervous tissue, with consequent extensive neuronal damage. The viral genome of the SARS-CoV was also found in the CSF of a patient with generalized convulsion [42]. In another patient with severe CNS symptoms who died for SARS, electronic microscopy on specimens of brain tissue, and genetic identification, proved the presence of the coronavirus. Moreover, pathological examination and immunohistochemistry showed neuronal necrosis, important glial cell alterations (hyperplasia), and CD68+ monocytes/macrophages and CD3+ T lymphocytes infiltration in the brain mesenchyme [43]. Finally, in another study, SARS genome sequences were found in the brain of all SARS autopsies ($n = 8$), and tissue damages (scattered red degeneration), mostly in the hypothalamus and cortex, were reported [11].

1.3.1.2 Pathogenesis of Direct SARS-CoV-2 Damage

Structurally, the viral genome is coated by spike (S) glycoprotein, envelope (E), membrane (M), and nucleocapsid (N) proteins. The viral RNA is organized in a single molecule of linear positive-sense (single-stranded RNA) of approximately 30 kb in size—the largest known RNA viruses—and with a 5′-cap structure and 3′-polyadenylated tail. The S protein is a trimeric glycoprotein formed by an ectodomain, a single-pass transmembrane anchor, and an intracellular tail. It is composed of two subunits (S1 and S2) and plays a key role in virus binding and entry into host cells. Homotrimers of S proteins compose the spikes on the viral surface, forming the typical virus crown. Interestingly, the S1 subunit contains the receptor-binding domain (RBD) that binds to the peptidase domain of ACE2 and, probably, to other proteins as well. The ACE2 is metalloproteinase ectoenzyme expressed mostly in the lower airway epithelial cells (alveolar type II cells, transient secretory cells, nasal ciliated, and secretory cells), upper olfactory neuroepithelium, and vascular endothelial cells, although it was also detected in almost all human organs [44]. For example, the enzyme is expressed in gastrointestinal cells, particularly enterocytes in the small intestine and colon, cardiac pericytes, cardiomyocytes, corneal epithelial cells, renal epithelial cells, bile duct cells, gallbladder epithelial cells, testicular Sertoli cells, and alveolar macrophages [45]. The S2 subunit, which is composed of a fusion peptide, a transmembrane domain, and a cytoplasmic domain, is highly conserved and works for producing viral membrane fusion.

This is the general pattern of interaction between coronavirus and host. Binding to S1 domains and fusion of membranes, because of the S2 subunit working, confer the specificity of the virus/host interaction. For instance, the virulence of the murine hepatitis virus (MHV), which is a neurotropic murine coronavirus, is critically dependent on the linkage with murine carcinoembryonic antigen-related cell adhesion molecule 1a (mCEACAM1a) for cell entry; thus, it can only infect murine cells.

ACE2 is one of the key enzymes in the renin–angiotensin system (RAS) that regulate blood pressure arterial, fluids, electrolyte balance, and systemic vascular resistance. In the lungs, activation of the local RAS can affect the pathogenesis of lung damage through multiple mechanisms, such as an increase in vascular permeability, and alterations of alveolar epithelial cells. Activation of the pulmonary RAS involves renin, the initial enzyme of the RAS activation cascade; renin splits angiotensinogen generating angiotensin I (Ang-I, a decapeptide hormone, inactive). The major function of ACE is to convert Ang-I to angiotensin II (Ang-II, an octapeptide hormone). Ang-II is a chief bioactive element of the RAS pathway and exerts its effects by binding to two types of receptors, Ang type 1 (AT1) and Ang type 2 (AT2). The AT1 receptor is predominant in the adult organism, whereas the AT2 type expression is mostly found in fetal tissues (cell differentiation processes) but decreases after birth. Activation of AT1 induces vasoconstriction, cardiac hypertrophy, and fibrosis. On the other hand, the AT2 receptor plays a protective effect against the overstimulation of AT1 and, thus, an increase of AT2 receptor expression was observed in pathological conditions, such as vascular injury, and congestive heart failure. Nevertheless, AT2 receptors are not always protective [46]. Since this subtype is implicated in pain modulation, it could play a role in the phenomenon of COVID-19-related pain. Remarkably, ACE2 is the homolog of ACE. The type 2 isoform removes the carboxy-terminal phenylalanine in Ang-II to form the heptapeptide angiotensin (Ang)-(1–7). This peptide is also active and can produce the opposite effect to that of Ang-II. Probably, it can play a role in the pathogenesis of the clinical manifestations of the disease, including those related to the altered nociception (see paragraph 1.5 Pain and COVID-19: The COVID-Pain Issue).

The ACE2/RAS pathway is also involved in non-catalytic functions such as intestinal neutral amino acid transport. Even these further actions could be important in the neurotoxicity mechanisms of the virus (see Sect. 1.3.4).

Of note, while SARS-CoV and SARS-CoV-2 bind both to the ACE2 "receptor," MERS-CoV used another entry anchor: the human dipeptidyl peptidase 4 (DPP4, also known as CD26). Since there is a high affinity between ACE2 and DPP4, it was postulated that particular mutations can enhance the DPP4-binding ability of SARS-CoV-2-S [47].

About the different pathogenicity of SARS-CoV and SARS-CoV-2, the latter shows structural properties that enable stronger binding to the ACE2 receptor and better capability at invading host cells [48]. In particular, the RBD is the most variable domain; it is decisive for the specificity of species. The SARS-CoV-2 RBD presents only a 40% amino acid identity with that of SARS-CoV. In particular, four of five key residues within the RBD of SARS-CoV-2 are mutated when compared with that of SARS-CoV. This is of great importance as RBD is fundamental in the pathogenesis of the infection. Thus, SARS-CoV-2-S domain binds to the ACE2 with a higher affinity (10- to 20-fold higher) than that of SARS-CoV. Considering this evidence, the logical inference is that SARS-CoV-2 could be more capable of infecting and damaging the CNS than SARS-CoV.

Another important difference that could explain the different pathogenicity of the two viruses is the presence of a polybasic furin-type cleavage site (RRAR^S) at the S1/S2 junction in the SARS-CoV-2-S protein but not in SARS-CoV [49]. Of note, similar sequences were demonstrated in the S proteins of many other pathogenic human viruses, such as Ebola, HIV-1, and certain remarkably virulent strains of avian influenza [50]. On the other hand, because there are no differences in ACE2 expression concerning gender, ages, and races, receptor binding is not the main factor in determining the severity of the disease [51].

As mentioned, the binding RBD-ACE2 is followed by the activation of the S protein. This process is mediated by different host proteases. They execute the cleavage of a polybasic sequence at the S1/S2 site. This protein processing allows the complete activity of the S2 domain and the fusion of the viral and cellular membranes. It was demonstrated that SARS-CoV-2 S is mainly processed by a plasma membrane-associated type II transmembrane serine protease (TMPRSS2) [52]. TMPRSS2 is highly expressed in epithelial tissues, including epithelial cells of the respiratory, gastrointestinal, and urogenital tract. The cleavage and fusion processes can be also performed through other host proteases including but not limited to the metallopeptidase domain 17 (ADAM17), the proprotein convertases furin (activates proprotein substrates in secretory pathway compartments), proteins such as vimentin and clathrin (involved in the binding and membrane fusion mechanisms), extracellular proteases such as elastase secreted by the neutrophils, and lysosomal proteases such cathepsin L and cathepsin B [53].

Subsequently, the virus entries into host cells, and viral replication begins with the translation of the replicase-polymerase gene and the assembly of the replication–transcription complex organized in double-membrane vesicles. Genomic regions that codify for structural proteins are thus transcribed and new virions are assembled and egress from the cell.

In summary, the RBD of the viral S1 subunit binds to the peptidase domain of ACE2 in the airway epithelial cells and other tissues. The binding is followed by the processing of the viral polybasic site (proteolytic priming of the virus-decorating spikes), the fusion of the viral and cell membranes, and the release of the viral genome into the host cytoplasm. Subsequently, there is viral replication through cellular machinery, viral assembly, and maturation via the Golgi endoplasmic reticulum, and finally, new viruses are released.

1.3.1.3 The Ligand–Receptor Interaction and "Postreceptorial Mechanisms" in Nervous Tissue

Since the cell tropism mainly depends on viral affinities for cellular/tissue "receptors," understanding which receptor(s) is(are) involved in the pathogenesis of COVID-19, and especially if different tissues have different binding elements, is mandatory. Mechanisms of neurotropism are based on this assumption.

As previously indicated, the ACE2 is the most studied SARS-CoV-2 host-cell receptor. It is widely expressed and, in the CNS, it can be found in most neuronal, glial elements, and endothelial cells. In a human cell-based platform (BrainSphere model), which was previously used for investigating Zika, Dengue, and HIV, and now adopted for studying SARS-CoV-2 neurotropism, it was firstly proved the replication of this coronavirus into the neural cells. Moreover, the authors illustrated that the phenomenon can be mediated by the ACE2 receptor, highly expressed in the model [54].

In addition to ACE2, other elements present in host cells must be considered for their role in facilitating virus entry. Proteases such as TMPRSS2, furin (ubiquitously expressed in endothelial cells and other target cells), and cathepsin L play a key role in viral pathogenicity. TMPRSS2 is probably the most studied of them. It can be an important element capable of conditioning organotropism. In the prostate tissue, for example, androgens can induce the expression of this protease and this finding may explain why men usually experience more severe forms of COVID-19 than women despite these latter are infected with the virus as frequently as men. Nevertheless, other factors such as the higher expression of ACE 2, and lifestyle (e.g., higher levels of smoking and drinking) can justify the greater vulnerability of men as compared to women. Concerning the role of TMPRSS2 in SARS-CoV-2 neurotropism, interesting findings came from preclinical investigations. Qiao et al. [55] showed that this serine protease is highly expressed in human and mouse brain cell lines, as well as in different murine brain regions. Moreover, the authors proved an important expression of CD147. Also termed as basigin, tumor collagenase stimulatory factor (TCSF), neurothelin, OX47, 5A11, or extracellular matrix metalloproteinase inducer (EMMPRIN), CD147 is a transmembrane glycoprotein that belongs to the immunoglobulin superfamily. In the CNS, it is expressed mostly in the hippocampus, prefrontal cortex, and amygdala, and exerts a paramount role in the homeostasis through regulatory and protective functions such as transport of nutrients, migration of inflammatory leukocytes, and induction of extracellular matrix. Furthermore, it takes part in intercellular recognition in several immunological processes and cellular differentiation events, in both neurons and glial cells [56]. On the other hand, its deregulation/upregulation is implicated in the pathogenesis of several CNS diseases such as Alzheimer's disease [57, 58], and multiple sclerosis, in CNS oncological processes, ischemic damage, and bacterial and virus infection [59]. These CD147-induced actions, mostly realize through the secretion of matrix metalloproteinases (MMPs), for example, from tumor cells or fibroblasts. Interestingly, the CD147-S protein binding seems to induce viral endocytosis and, probably, there could be a different mechanism than the typical RBD-ACE2 binding [60]. Research must prove whether this interaction, at least in part, can explain the neurotropic phenomenon of SARS-CoV-2. However, different lines of evidence must necessarily be considered. Previous studies in an animal model of experimental autoimmune encephalomyelitis, for example, suggested that CD147 acts as a regulator of leukocyte transmigration into the CNS [61]. Since leukocytes can cross the endothelial basement membrane but require proteases such as MMPs to transmigrate the glia limitans, it could be assumed that CD147 activation facilitates the BBB injury by stimulating leukocyte transmigration via MMPs secretion.

Other factors are probably involved in ACE2-mediated SARS-CoV-2 infection and determine the tropism of the virus. The furin-induced proteolytic cleavage of RRAR^S sequence exposes a conserved C-terminal sequence in the S protein. This pattern is indicated as RXXROH—in particular, R is arginine (or lysine) and X is any amino acid—and structures a C-end rule (CendR) that bind to and activate neuropilin (NRP1 and NRP2) receptors at the cell surface. Cantuti-Castelvetri et al. [62] demonstrated that NRP1 can highly potentiate SARS-CoV-2 infectivity. Moreover, this effect was effectively blocked by a monoclonal blocking antibody against NRP1. In one of their fascinating experiments, the same authors administered nanoparticles coated with SARS-CoV-2 S–derived CendR peptides—one miming SARS-2 S protein after furin cleavage able to bind NRP1, and another one which reduced NRP1 binding (control)—into cultured cells expressing NRP1, olfactory epithelium, and the CNS of anesthetized adult mice. Six hours after administration, compared to control, they proved a significant uptake of the miming nanoparticles into the cells, olfactory epithelium, as well as into neurons, and blood vessels of the cortex. The authors demonstrated the role of NP1 in SARS-CoV-2 pathogenicity.

1.3.2 Mechanisms of Diffusion Towards the Nervous Tissue

As demonstrated for other HCoVs, the SARS-CoV-2 virus could reach the CNS routes by the following two routes:

- Hematogenous route.
- Nervous spreading.

According to the hematogenous pathway, the virus can reach CNS/PNS via the blood route during the viremia. On the other hand, the nervous spreading could involve some cranial nerves, such as the olfactory nerve, the trigeminal nerve, the glossopharyngeal nerve, and the vagus. The general scheme of the nerve spreading provides a retrograde transport of the virus, up to the brain.

1.3.2.1 The Hematogenous Route

Although the respiratory system is the primary route used by SARS-CoV-2, it could be not the only one. The viral transmission occurs through droplets secreted by the patient during coughing, sneezing, breathing, and even normal speech. The Type II alveolar epithelial cells that express high concentrations of ACE2 are the respiratory gate. Alternatively, the virus can use gastrointestinal access through the ACE2 receptor [63]. Other potential SARS-CoV-2 transmission routes must be well-investigated; for example, the conjunctival route through infectious tears was demonstrated in rhesus macaques [64].

Whatever the route, the virus reaches the circulation and projects itself towards different organs and tissues, including the CNS. Here, the ligand coupling seems to occur at the endothelial cells and, and even in this case, the ACE2 plays a fundamental role. In this regard, in an autopsy investigation, Paniz-Mondolfi et al. [65] reported the presence of SARS-CoV-2 in capillary endothelial cells in neural tissue (frontal lobe) collected from a COVID-19 patient. This finding may support the hematogenous-endothelial neuroinvasion mechanism. This mechanism involves the overcoming of the BBB filter—composed of endothelial cells of the capillary wall, astrocyte end-feet ensheathing the capillary, and pericytes embedded in the capillary basement membrane—which undergoes a more or less localized process of destruction. This injury is secondary to the direct viral attack and, in turn, to the inflammatory phenomena triggered by the activation of local defense mechanisms. From this point of view, in the case of the primary neurotropism of SARS-CoV-2, the damage to the BBB differs from that produced by cytokines. In this latter case, indeed, the BBB involvement is more diffuse as it can encompass multiple brain areas. Furthermore, the integrity of the BBB is mainly undermined by the triggering of neuroinflammation rather than by the viral attack.

The major task of BBB is to create a protective front for preventing the passage of substances/pathogens from the arterial blood into the cerebral extracellular fluid, reaching and, finally, damaging the nervous tissue. While preclinical studies on mice highlighted that the isolated S1 subunit can cross the entire thickness of the BBB [66], this structure offers a barrier to viral penetration into the CNS. The BBB is not the only brain barrier; the other barrier is the blood-cerebrospinal fluid barrier (BCSFB) that prevents the passage of substances/pathogens from the cerebral capillaries to the CSF at the level of the choroid plexuses. BCSFB is made up of the capillary endothelium and the epithelium of the choroid plexus. Once this barrier is overcome, a substance or a pathogen spreads directly into the CSF and from there it could reach the extracellular fluid of the nervous tissue. As evidence of the existence of this potential entry route, there is the finding of the viral genome (SARS-CoV-2 mRNA) in the CSF of a patient suffering from neurological manifestations of COVID-19 [37]. Nevertheless, further proofs are needed to confirm this pathway.

1.3.2.2 The Neurogenic Pathway

In line with many other neuroinvasive viruses [67], the gateway used by the SARS-CoV-2 to enter into the CNS is mainly represented by the olfactory system (Fig. 1.2). This data may explain important clinical aspects of the disease. As previously reported, alterations in smell are demonstrated in about a quarter of patients with COVID-19; however, clinical studies conducted with the aid of ad hoc tests were able to identify hyposmia in up to 80% of patients [68]. It showed that this finding is underestimated. Therefore, it was postulated that olfactory receptor neurons (ORNs) and the olfactory system could represent a portal of entry for neuroinvasion by HCoVs.

The olfactory system is composed of the ORNs, the olfactory bulb (OB) which is a processing station, and the primary olfactory cortex which is located on the inferior surface of the temporal lobe. ORNs are bipolar neurons that are activated when airborne molecules in inspired air bind to olfactory receptors expressed on their cilia (dendrites). These sensorial neurons are found high inside the nasal vault in the olfactory epithelium. The latter is placed on the lower surface of the

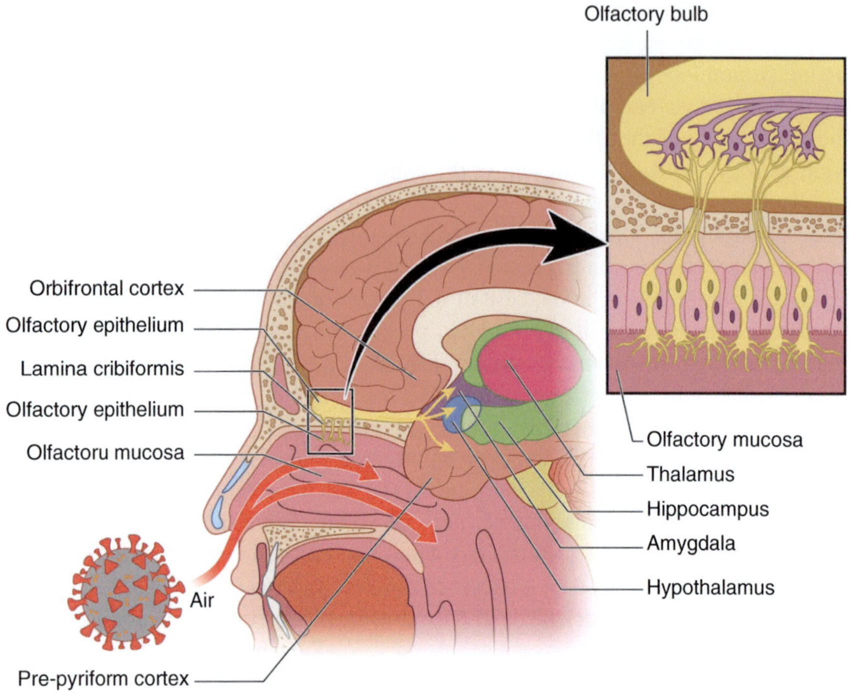

Fig. 1.2 The entry way of the olfactory system. The system is composed of receptor neurons (bipolar sensory neurons found in the epithelium of the nasal vault), olfactory bulb, and primary olfactory cortex (located inferiorly in the temporal lobe). The axons of the receptor neurons synapse with neurons of the olfactory bulb in the cribriform lamina [second neurons (mitral and tufted cells) of the olfactory pathway]. They project to the anterior olfactory nucleus, the olfactory tubercle, the prepyriform cortex, and the amygdala, which together form the olfactory cortex. From here other projections start towards the limbic system of the brain (emotions and memories), hypothalamus (eating and nutrition), and thalamus (sensory processing)

cribriform lamina of the ethmoid bone, on the medial surface of the upper and middle turbinates, and the upper nasal septum. The axon extensions of the ORNs aggregate into fascicles and cross the small foramina in the cribriform plate. Here, the axons synapse in intricate neural masses (glomeruli) in the OB. Each ORN axon innervates only a single glomerulus. The OB contains the second neurons (mitral and tufted cells) of the olfactory pathway and processes the stimuli through the action of interneurons, granular cells, and periglomerular cells. Axons emerge from the OB to form the lateral olfactory tract, which subsequently projects to the anterior olfactory nucleus, the olfactory tubercle, the prepyriform cortex, and the amygdala, which are known collectively as the olfactory cortex. From these areas, multiple synaptic circuits develop. Notably, elements of the olfactory cortex are part of the limbic system of the brain (emotions and memories). Moreover, there are projections to the hypothalamus (eating and nutrition) and thalamus (sensory processing). The latter refers to other brain areas. From the thalamus, for example,

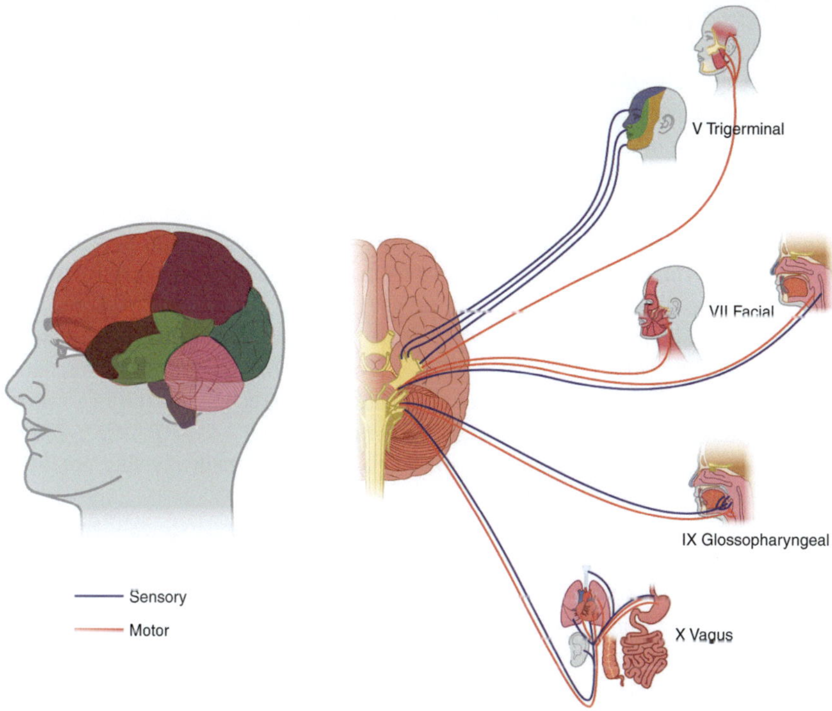

Fig. 1.3 Potential retrograde pathways followed by the virus to access the CNS. The pathway involves some cranial nerves such as the trigeminal nerve (III), facial nerve (VII), glossopharyngeal nerve (IX), and vagus nerve (X)

projections develop to associative areas of the orbitofrontal neocortex for the conscious perception of the olfactory sensation.

Since the olfactory epithelium is exposed to multiple insults (biological, chemical, traumatic) and can be continuously damaged, a regeneration mechanism is expected. In the olfactory epithelium, basal cells act as neuronal stem cells, capable of restoring or regenerating the lost olfactory epithelial cells. The axon then regenerates and gets back in contact with the OB. The axons are surrounded by glial cells that ensure the regeneration of these axons, acting as a "guide" and allowing them to reach their original target again. The regeneration cycle lasts about a month.

The olfactory system is not the only neurogenic gate the virus can use, and it is not the only nervous structure to be exposed to viral damage (Fig. 1.3). Moreover, it must be considered that several factors such as aging are associated with reduced ACE2 expression and, more importantly, the degeneration of ORNs [69]. Concerning gates other than that of the OS, the respiratory mucosa of the nasal cavity is innervated by the trigeminal nerve. It is the fifth paired cranial nerve that originates from three sensory nuclei (mesencephalic, principal sensory, spinal nuclei of the trigeminal nerve) and one motor nucleus (motor nucleus of the trigeminal nerve) extending from the midbrain to the medulla. Thus, it represents another hypothetical way for the centripetal routing of the SARS-CoV-2. In early studies, it was proved that MHV can spread into the CNS via the neuronal circuit of the trigeminal nerve [70]. This pathway is also used by other respiratory viruses such as the respiratory syncytial virus, and influenza virus [71].

Besides alterations in smell, patients with COVID-19 may experience alterations in taste in terms of hypogeusia or dysgeusia. Interestingly, this sense is conveyed via three cranial nerves, the facial nerve (VII), the glossopharyngeal nerve (IX), and the vagus nerve (X). The first processing station of the sensation is the nucleus of the solitary tract, which is found in the brainstem. Subsequently, the information is conveyed to the thalamus. Consequently, COVID-19-induced taste alterations can be produced by damage affecting one of these cranial nerves. Of note, because in the brainstem the nucleus of the tract solitary is close to the respiratory center, damage caused by the virus that spreads along the taste pathway could result in a neurogenic respiratory alteration. Although genomic material of SARS-CoV-2 was detected in a patient with conjunctivitis [72], the ocular pathway has not been clearly demonstrated so far.

Inconclusive data exists on the intracellular (intraneural) and extracellular (extraneural) propagation of SARS-CoV-2. Some information can be gleaned from previous studies on HCoVs. In a mouse model and neuronal cell cultures, Dubé et al. [73] showed the axonal transport of the HCoV OC43 within several areas of the brain, such as the hippocampus, diencephalon, and cortex, and this pathway enabled HCoV OC43 neuron-to-neuron propagation. In turn, a synaptic transfer is performed. Since it was previously demonstrated for other HCoVs, the synaptic transfer mechanism is not exclusive to SARS-CoV-2. In 2012, Li et al. [74] carried out interesting experiments in rats. They performed peripheral inoculation of the HEV coronavirus in the animals and found an extensive amount of HEV antigen in the cell bodies of sensory neurons (dorsal root ganglia (DRG) neurons). The authors also proved the replication and assembly of HEV in the cytoplasm of these neurons and that the exit process of the virus is realized mainly by the large smooth-surfaced vesicle-mediated pathway. Another potential mechanism for viral propagation is the passive diffusion of released viral particles. Probably, SARS-CoV-2 and other coronaviruses use both strategies including passive diffusion of released viral particles and axonal transport through kinesins, dynein, and motor proteins, for performing their propagation.

In summary, viruses may enter through the gate of the olfactory system or other neurogenic gates such as the trigeminal route and, in turn, are probably transferred to the CNS via a synapse-connected route or through the trans-neuronal propagation. Whatever the mechanism, via neuronal retrograde transport, SARS-CoV-2 might reach cortical and subcortical brain areas, as well as the brainstem, and the spinal cord.

1.3.2.3 Other Possible Routes

Besides the hematogenous pathway, which involves binding with the endothelial cells of the BBB, and the centripetal neurogenic pathways, other routes used for viral access to the nervous tissue may exist. In this regard, Lima et al. [75], based on the neuroinvasive behavior of known HCoVs, and on the evidence that these viruses can infect bloodstream leukocytes, postulated the "trojan horse" mechanism of SARS-CoV-2. In other words, as proposed for human immunodeficiency virus (HIV) [76], the virus could reach the SNC through infected immune circulating cells. This route can be viewed as a variant of the "classic" hematogenous route and presupposes a particular and poorly investigated receptor-independent entry instead that the classic receptor-mediated endocytosis mechanism.

The lymphatic pathway is a very fascinating hypothesis although completely to be verified. Until recently, it was believed that the brain did not have the classic lymphatic vessels. The so-called glymphatic system represents a system that allows CNS perfusion by the CSF and interstitial fluid. Since this system encompasses olfactory/cervical lymphatic vessels, it could contribute to a direct entry of the SARS-CoV-2 to the brain. As proof of this potential mechanism of viral spreading, it was histologically proved that SARS-CoV-2 can infect lymph endothelial cells, disseminating to the nasal cavity from cervical lymph nodes and, finally, reaching the brain glymphatic system [77].

1.3.3 Immune-Mediated Neurological Processes

Many of the clinical manifestations of neuro-COVID can be explained through an immune-mediated mechanism. For instance, molecular mimicry between viral proteins and proteins on peripheral nerves leading to autoantibody-mediated damage to myelin or axons may explain the pathogenesis of Guillain-Barré syndrome. However, in immune-mediated processes, an important role is mostly played by systemic responses through massive release of cytokines and macrophage activation.

1.3.3.1 Cytokine Storm

Besides the direct neurotoxic effect, SARS-CoV-2 can produce neurological damages through the activation of an excessive immune response. This exuberant immune-mediated inflammation is a cornerstone of a cascade of events that culminates in the development of the various clinical manifestations of COVID-19. The acute respiratory distress syndrome (ARDS), for instance, is produced by a direct viral attack to pulmonary and endothelium cells, combined with immune-mediated inflammation with dysfunctional coagulation.

The mechanism of the coronavirus-induced neuroinflammation needs to be better elucidated. Although many pieces of the puzzle must be still assembled, the complex chain of events that produces the immune-mediated damage is progressively enriched with new scientific findings. A key concept is the dysregulation in the production of soluble immune mediators. This phenomenon involves the activation and inhibition of different immune cell subtypes and, consequently, a dysregulation between the production of mediators with anti-inflammatory action and other deleterious substances that induce the recall of further cellular elements, with endothelial damage, and alteration of the microcirculation. This complex phenomenon is termed "cytokine storm." It is expressed as a high release of proinflammatory cytokines such as interleukin-6 (IL-6), tumor necrosis factor α (TNF-α), IL-1β, IL-8, IL-12, and IL-18, as well as interferon (IFN) gamma inducible protein (IP10; also termed as motif chemokine ligand 10, CXCL10), macrophage inflammatory protein 1A (MIP1A), and monocyte chemoattractant protein 1 (MCP1) [78].

In COVID-19, the processes that trigger the immune responses against the virus are, at least partly, unknown and much data has been translated from SARS research. The aberrant virus-induced dysregulation of the immunologic response, indeed, was also observed during the SARS and MERS outbreaks. For instance, it was shown that SARS-CoV is recognized by the toll-like receptors (TLR), especially TLR3 and TLR4. TLRs are a class of single-pass, non-catalytic transmembrane receptors mainly expressed on the membrane of sentinel cells such as macrophages and dendritic cells. They play a key role in the defense of the organism, in particular in innate immunity. The binding of SARS-CoV-2 to the TLRs induces the release of pro-IL-1β which is cleaved into the active mature IL-1β. The latter mediates lung inflammation through the activation of the inflammasome [79]. Furthermore, within the neuroimmune responses, the hyperactivation of the P2X7 receptor could play an important role. These receptors are ATP-gated ion channels extensively found in the CNS. Of note, mental disorders and behavioral alterations can follow virus-induced neuroimmune processes characterized by oxygen species (ROS) formation, and glutamate release [80]. Also in this case the process would be configured through the activation of inflammasomes. They are cytosolic multiprotein oligomers (inflammasomes complexes) of the innate immune system that induce activation of inflammatory responses through cleavage, maturation, and secretion of proinflammatory cytokines IL-1β and IL-18 [81].

Since the description of lung damage through cytokine storm is outside the scope of this chapter, it seems appropriate to focus the reader's attention on the possible intersection between the COVID-19-induced deregulated immune response and the CNS alterations.

In addition to IL-1β, other immune mediators that are aberrantly produced in response to SARS-CoV-2 can lead to neurotoxicity. Of those, IL-1β, IL-6, IP10, and TNFα are the proinflammatory cytokines with the greater ability to induce tissue injury in several organs, including the CNS. However, the list of proinflammatory substances triggered by the infection is particularly long and includes other ILs such as IL-12 p40, IL-20, and IL-33, and the gamma-interferon-inducible protein Ifi-16 (Ifi-16). In a mouse model, most of these proinflammatory cytokines and the role of astrocytes and microglia were demonstrated [82]. Other investigators showed that primary glial cell cultures exposed to coronavirus can secrete a substantial amount of several proinflammatory cytokines, especially IL-15, IL-6, and TNFα [71].

Thus, several pathways are involved in the virus-induced tissue damage. This aberrant activation of inflammatory and prothrombotic pathways leads to further cellular recruitment with chemo-attraction of macrophages, and cellular stress, mostly resulting from activated ROS. In particular, coagulopathy plays a key role in the mechanisms of neurotoxicity. The COVID-19-associated coagulopathy is a complex phenomenon. It reflects microthrombi formation secondary to endothelial

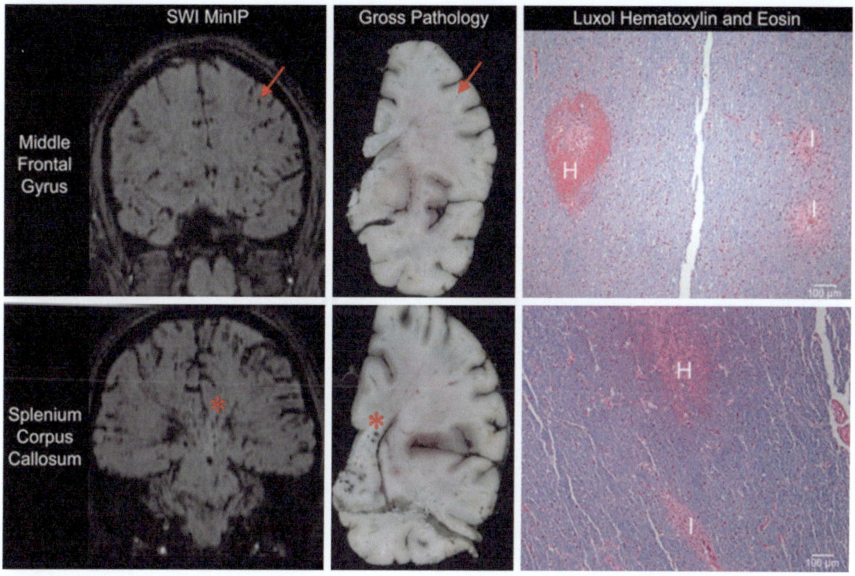

Fig. 1.4 Radiologic-pathologic correlations of the microvascular lesions. Punctate hypointense foci at the middle frontal gyrus (red arrow) and splenium of the corpus callosum (asterisk) are indicated (MRI Susceptibility weighted minimum-intensity projection images). The microscopy analysis shows corresponding lesions in coronal tissue slabs and eosin. They are characterized by microhemorrhages (H) and microscopic ischemic lesions (I). From Conklin J, et al. J Neurol Sci (2021) 421:117308 © Elsevier with permission

cell inflammation combined with deregulated immune reaction and cytokines release (Fig. 1.4).

This cascade produces hypercoagulability with venous thromboembolism and arterial occlusion [83]. However, the damage can also concern vessels of smaller caliber. As suggested by neuroimaging investigations, multifocal microvascular hemorrhagic and ischemic lesions in the subcortical and deep white matter can underlie many neurological manifestations of the disease (Fig. 1.5).

The pathophysiology of the cytokine storm (or cytokine release syndrome, CRS), and its effects on the nervous tissue, has been particularly studied for addressing toxicity associated with chimeric antigen receptor (CAR) T cell therapy in patients with onco-hematological malignancies. CAR-T represents the first form of gene therapy approved for the treatment of refractory and relapsing onco-hematological diseases such as acute lymphoblastic leukemia in children and young adults, and some aggressive forms of non-Hodgkin lymphoma. It was proved that IL-1β and IL-6 are both extensively implicated in neurotoxicity after CAR-T treatment [84]. These cytokines, for example, have detrimental effects on endothelial function and can provoke a BBB breakdown. There is also BCSFB damage. It possibly reflects enhanced permeability and increased levels of multiple cytokines in the CSF [85]. Given these premises, in the early stages of the pandemic, it was suggested that agents directed against the deleterious cytokines could be used as therapeutic agents

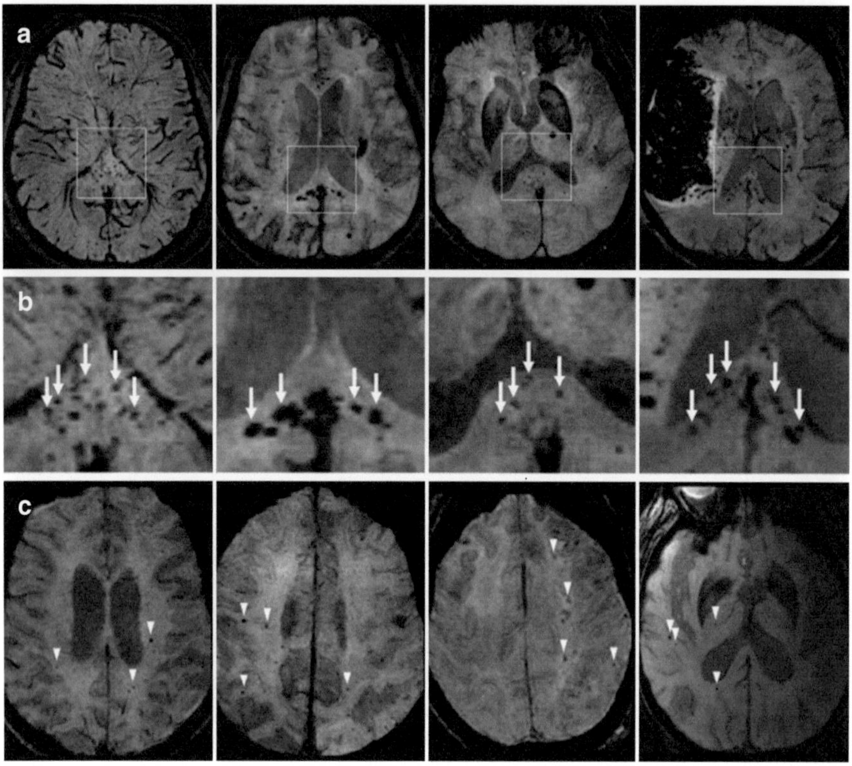

Fig. 1.5 Microvascular damage. RMI susceptibility weighted imaging (SWI) in four critically ill COVID-19 patients (**a**). Magnification views of the splenium of the corpus callosum for each patient (**b**) (arrows). Diffuse SWI lesions (arrowheads) involving the subcortical, periventricular and deep white matter, without involvement of the corpus callosum (**c**). From Conklin J, et al. J Neurol Sci (2021) 421:117308 © Elsevier with permission

in COVID-19. Consequently, tocilizumab, a humanized IgG1 monoclonal antibody, directed against the IL-6 receptor, and anakinra, a recombinant IL-1 receptor antagonist, were extensively tested [18].

1.3.3.2 Microglial Activation and Blood–Brain Barrier Damage

The underlying pathophysiology of acute neuro-COVID processes is probably different from that involving long-term effects. While many acute events, such as vascular ones, presuppose extensive damage where the vascular component is predominant, neuroinflammation plays a fundamental role in chronic events. In this context, alterations of the BBB are fundamental in the mechanisms of nervous tissue damage. Since many cytokines can easily cross the BBB to affect CNS function, lesions to the BBB are secondary to the effect of the neuroinflammation development.

Activation of microglia is a hallmark of all these processes. Microglia are the resident immune cells of the CNS. Under steady-state conditions, these cells live in a “resting” state and interact with the cell surface and soluble factors from surrounding cells. Exposure to pathogen-associated molecular patterns and/or endogenous damage-associated molecular patterns, and removal of the immune-suppressive signals, provokes microglia activation. Notably, depending on the signals in the surrounding environment, these activated cells can show different phenotypes. In particular, because it promotes a proinflammatory response, the M1 phenotype is initially present succeeding an insult. Subsequently, the response is shifted to be anti-inflammatory which is mediated by M2 microglia. This is a simplistic but didactic scheme. Probably, there is a range of microglial activation states that span from the M1 to M2 phenotypes, and each phenotype can show different markers, secrete peculiar compounds, and exhibit distinctive functions.

On these premises, the dynamics of long-COVID neurocognitive problems can be like those described in other neuroinflammation-based processes such as delirium [86], postoperative cognitive dysfunction [87], and chemotherapy-related cognitive impairment [88]. Moreover, the neuroinflammatory responses followed by hemorrhagic lesions and neuronal impairment have been extensively illustrated in psychiatric disorders and neurodegenerative diseases [89]. The general scheme provides that neuroinflammation due to several causes is expressed as a loop with microglial activation (M2 microglia), increased oxidative stress activation, microcircle alterations, and progressive BBB damage. It leads to further recruitment of peripheral immune cells into the brain and BBB permeability. The effects are aberrant neuronal signaling and structural alterations in several brain regions (e.g., hippocampus, striatum, medial prefrontal cortex, and gyrus cinguli).

The issue of neuroinflammation opens other scenarios. For example, the SARS-CoV-2 infection could trigger and/or worse underlying brain diseases. Individuals with CNS disorders featuring neuroimmune activation such as Parkinson’s and Alzheimer’s disease may be more prone to coronavirus infection. In these patients, indeed, the increased BBB permeability could facilitate SARS-CoV-2 neuroinvasion. In the same way, the infection can precipitate the degenerative pathology, accelerating the fall of the neurocognitive trajectory. Further research and epidemiological studies must prove these assumptions.

Overlapping processes may be possible and complicate the pathogenic cascade. As previously demonstrated for other viruses such as West Nile virus, and Japanese encephalitis virus, in an advanced stage of the disease, the cytokine storm could cause extensive damage to the tight junctions of the BBB. It can favor the triggering of viral neurotropism and the entry into the CNS [90, 91]. In other words, the infection activates the immune system which, when deregulated, induces a cumbersome response that results in the cytokine storm; consequently, more or less extensive damage is produced to the integrity of the BBB and/or BCSFB and this process opens the access routes of the CNS to the virus increasing its uptake into the brain. At this point, the virus carries out its virulence strategies. Co-factors such as the ARDS-induced hypoxia combined or not with the organ damage, the adopted invasive therapies, and co-infections may amplify or precipitate the cascade.

1.3.4 Gut–Brain Axis Involvement

In the uncertainties on precise mechanisms for neuro-COVID, all hypotheses need to be discussed. A fascinating supposition relates the intestinal organotropism of the virus to the triggering of neurological symptomatology. Neurological alterations would be induced by an alteration of the gut–brain axis, secondary to direct viral damage to intestinal cells and microbiota alterations [92]. The gut–brain axis works by maintaining homeostasis in terms of a proper functioning of the digestive tract. It also regulates other functions of the immune system and brain activities. This pathway is so important that its impairments (dysbiosis) are implicated in the pathogenesis of functional gastrointestinal processes like irritable bowel syndrome, and several psychiatric, neurodevelopmental, age-related, and neurodegenerative disorders.

In brief, there is bidirectional communication between microbiota and the brain. This communication is obtained via neural, endocrine, immune, and humoral links. Microbial metabolites such as short-chain fatty acids, branched-chain amino acids, and peptidoglycans, as well as choline metabolites, lactate, and vitamins, are involved in this complex functional system. Again, the enteric nervous system and the vagus nerve, the spinal cord, the autonomic nervous system, and the hypothalamic pituitary adrenal axis compose the neural side of the axis.

At least hypothetically, the axis could be involved in the pathogenesis of the neuro-COVID. In the intestines, ACE2 receptors work as co-receptors for the intake of nutrients including amino acids and regulate the development of gut microbiota and innate immunity mechanisms. Thus, intestinal organotropism of SARS-CoV-2 can underlie the gastrointestinal symptoms of the disease such as diarrhea, vomiting, nausea, abdominal pain. Cytokine-induced mechanisms, via IL-6, TNFα, and other proinflammatory molecules, can be implicated in the pathogenic cascade which also includes opportunistic infections [93]. These processes can predispose to psychiatric, or neurocognitive manifestations of COVID-19 such as depression, delirium, and confusion. The hypothesized mechanisms include reduction in the production of 5-hydroxytyphtophan (serotonin) and catecholamines (because of reduced intake of the precursor tryptophan), reduced availability of metabolites produced by the normal bacterial flora, and alteration of the vagus nerve centripetal transmission. The latter is physiologically projected to several brain areas such as the solitary nucleus, thalamus, hypothalamus, locus coeruleus, amygdala, and periaqueductal gray (PAG). The hypothalamic–pituitary–adrenal axis can be also involved. Therefore, most important functions can be impaired.

The potential involvement of the gut–brain axis shows very interesting pathogenic presupposes. However, although some symptoms such as delirium (excessive dopamine availability), confusion (proinflammatory state), and abdominal pain (functional alteration of the endogenous opioid system and PAG) may find a fairly plausible explanation, for other clinical manifestations, such as those from acute damage (sensory alterations), the role of the axis is difficult to be explained. They are probably provoked by direct and/or indirect viral injury. Overlapping processes cannot be excluded and alterations of the axis between the intestine and the brain can intersect with different pathogenic mechanisms responsible for neurological damage.

1.3.5 Effects of Multiorgan Dysfunction

This group of pathogenetic mechanisms does not foresee direct viral damage, nor the activation of a cascade of events that triggered by the virus induces neurotoxicity through the host inflammatory response phase of the disease.

Hypoxia and organ damage, invasive therapies, and co-infections amplify the cascade of events that determine neurotoxicity. In other words, neurological complications represent an epiphenomenon of a multisystem disease. For example, electrolytes disturbances can induce seizures. Moreover, the binding of the virus to ACE2 receptors can produce a fluctuation of blood pressure and weakening of the endothelial layer, leading to a dysfunction of cerebral autoregulation and altered BBB function with hypoperfusion of the posterior circulation. This process is probably underlined to the posterior reversible encephalopathy syndrome featuring altered consciousness, seizures, headaches, and visual disturbances. Furthermore, delirium or decreased level of consciousness up to coma with or without seizures and extrapyramidal signs can be explained as acute encephalopathy due to hypoxia and alteration of neurotransmitters.

1.4 Potential Mechanisms for Long-Term Neurotoxicity

A special chapter of the neuro-COVID problem concerns the possibility that the infection and/or neuroinflammatory processes can be able to accelerate or precipitate brain aging phenomena, neurovascular coupling, and age-related or other underlying neurodegenerative disorders. This aspect is of crucial importance and concerns the possible long-term complications in COVID-19-survivors.

For this reason, pathophysiology has the hard task to find a linkage between the hitherto known aspects of the disease and the common mechanisms of neurodegeneration. In addition, while the clinical-epidemiological research must provide precise data on the phenomenon, it is necessary to underline how COVID-19-survivors need accurate monitoring that must include a careful neurocognitive follow-up.

Several mechanisms need to be considered for explaining the potential virus-induced acceleration of neurodegenerative processes. As previously addressed, immune-mediated neurological processes with microglial activation and BBB impairment can play a key role. Nevertheless, it must be considered that rather than direct or indirect viral damage, neurodegeneration appears more likely to be produced by the disease as a whole. Consequently, it would be more appropriate to refer to COVID-19-induced neurodegeneration [94].

Potential mechanisms for long-term cognitive alterations are manifold (Table 1.1). Changes in the neurocardiac axis are one of the putative mechanisms.

Table 1.1 Potential mechanisms for long-term neurotoxicity

Process	Mechanism(s)
Neurocardiac axis	Alteration in the axis can induce decreased BDNF levels and an increased susceptible of the CNS to the cellular damage
Neurovascular damage	Cytokines-induced BBB damages in key associative areas
Demyelination	Immune-mediated demyelination Impairment of oligodendrocyte progenitor cells
Neurodegeneration	Neuroinflammation through cytokines production, BBB damage, cells recruitments (microglial activation), further oxidative stress, and neurotransmission alterations in particular brain regions
Cellular senescence	Virus-induced senescence brain cells (oligodendrocytes and astrocytes) can produce proinflammatory cytokines, maintaining the neuroinflammation

Abbreviations: *BDNF* brain-derived neurotropic factor, *CNS* central nervous system, *BBB* blood–brain barrier

This axis concerns a communication system that links the cardiovascular and nervous systems aimed at maintaining healthy cardiac contraction. It works through the sympathetic and parasympathetic outflow and the action of the brain-derived neurotropic factor (BDNF). Also called abrineurin, this protein is closely related to the nerve growth factor. It has an important role in vasculogenesis, neurogenesis, axonal sprouting, and memory consolidation. It was demonstrated a decline of BDNF in aging and its role in precipitating the cognitive decline [95]. During the COVID-19, any alteration in the axis (e.g., due to cardiomyocytes damage) can provoke decreased BDNF expression and, in turn, an increased susceptibility of the nervous tissues to the cellular damage.

As previously mentioned regarding the hematogenous pathway of diffusion of SARS-CoV-2, the virus can bind to the ACE2 of the endothelium of cerebral vessels. These cells, together with neurons, astrocytes, vascular smooth muscle cells, and pericytes, combine to form the BBB structure. Therefore, an alteration of the BBB—eventually produced by the proinflammatory systemic state— in addition to opening a way of access to viral invasion (an eventuality yet to be verified), creates a substantial alteration of neuronal functioning with alterations of the microcirculation and loss of filter function towards neurotoxic agents. All these phenomena, when involving key associative areas, predispose and/or accelerate the cognitive decline typical of aging.

Demyelination is another potential mechanism underlying long-term damage in the nervous tissue. As Desforges et al. [12] demonstrated, the genome of HCoVs was isolated in brain specimens set up at autopsy of individuals affected by neurodegenerative diseases. Previously, Lane et al. [17] conducted investigations on the pathogenesis of murine coronavirus infection of the CNS and highlighted that viral persistence in oligodendrocytes may induce immune-mediated demyelination. Probably, the extend of the clinical manifestations depends on the degree of cell impairment and by the differentiation capability of oligodendrocyte progenitor cells. Of note, ACE2 was also found in these latter cells [45].

The infection-induced neuroinflammation is another issue to be addressed for explaining the late-onset neuro-COVID. Nevertheless, the cascade involving cytokine production, BBB damage, cells recruitment (microglial activation), and finally further oxidative stress with neurotransmission problems in particular brain regions must be well elucidated. On these bases, it was hypnotized that chronic-neuro-COVID could be linked to an ongoing low-grade inflammatory response and/or degeneration of functional neuronal and glial cells, while the vascular occlusion seems mostly involved in the acute phase of the disease [96]. Notably, in a study that compared the serum of patients 40–45 days after the infection to that of healthcare workers without infection, persistence of the inflammatory response and mitochondrial stress was found [97].

Finally, a virus-induced senescence mechanism that leads to a reduced capacity to respond to differentiation and apoptotic stimuli cannot be excluded. Senescence brain cells including oligodendrocytes and astrocytes can produce proinflammatory cytokines, maintaining the neuroinflammation process.

1.5 Pain and COVID-19: The COVID-Pain Issue

In the context of the neurological manifestations of COVID-19, pain is a special problem [98]. Painful issues can be schematically divided into two types:

- COVID-19-associated acute pain conditions.
- Long-term painful clinical manifestations.

The acute forms regard the acute course of the disease; on the other hand, the long-term manifestations must be framed as COVID-19 outcomes and are encompassed in the long-COVID issue. These two sets present pathophysiological, clinical, prognostic, and health care differences. Even in this case, however, the distinction has mainly narrative purposes. The hypothesized mechanisms—for example, an imbalance in the production of cytokines with opposite action in nociception—could affect the mechanisms of acute pain but, at the same time, they can also be responsible for the genesis of chronic pain processes (Fig. 1.6).

1.5.1 Acute Clinical Manifestations

In terms of pathophysiology, an interpretation for understanding the COVID-19-associated acute pain clinical manifestations is the ACE2/RAS pathway and its variable expression in key areas of nociception. Through the action of different angiotensinogen cleavage products that act as neurotransmitters and/or neuromodulators, and their impact on particular receptors and post-receptor pathways, complex neuromodulation in the spinal transmission of nociceptive information is performed. Theoretically, the SARS-CoV-2 could impact these mechanisms by altering the balance between the neuromodulation systems of nociception.

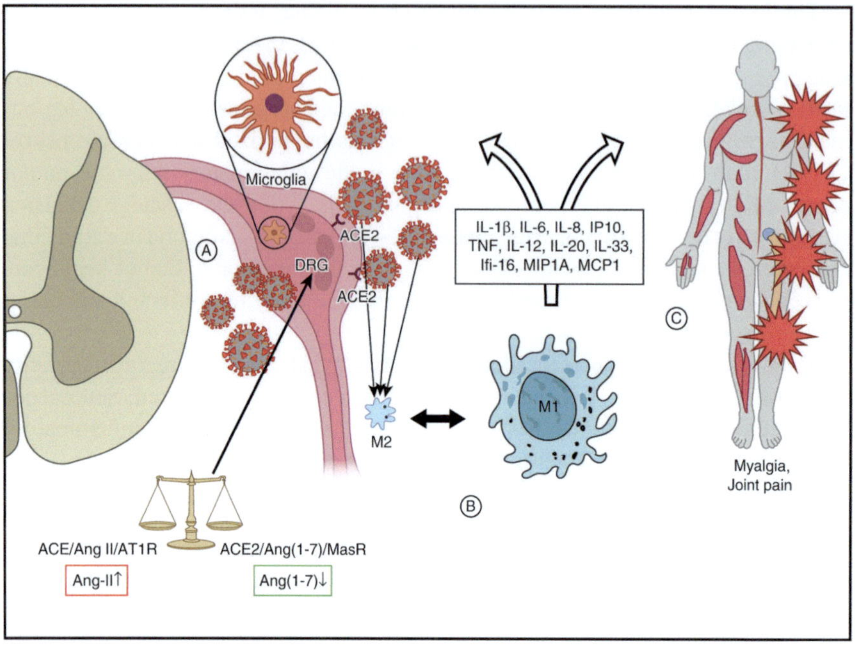

Fig. 1.6 Potential mechanisms of COVID-pain. (**a**) ACE2/RAS pathway and the direct virus-induced damage. Within the RAS, the virus/receptor (ACE2) interaction involves unbalance of the ACE/Ang II/AT1R and the ACE2/Ang-(1–7)/MasR axes with down-regulation of ACE2 levels on cell surfaces, Ang-II accumulation, and impairment of the anti-nociceptive Ang-(1-7) pathway. (**b**) Macrophage activation. Macrophages and other immune cells can stimulate the production of inflammatory mediators (e.g., IL-1β, TNF, and bradykinins). These processes can facilitate the sensory cells injury and can lead to chronic pain through sensitization/activation mechanisms. (**c**) The exuberant immune-mediated inflammation. It can induce widespread myalgia and joint pain via peripheral and central mechanisms. Disease-related and predisposing factors contribute to the determinism of the damage. Abbreviation: RAS, renin–angiotensin system; ACE2, angiotensin-converting enzyme 2; Ang, angiotensin; AT1R, angiotensin 1 receptor; MasR, Mas receptor; IL, interleukin; TNF, tumor necrosis factor

Preclinical studies in mice showed that the ACE2 is expressed in neurons and microglia (but not astrocytes) in the DRG [99]. The activation of AT1 receptors leads to nociception phenomena through the phosphorylation of p38 mitogen-activated protein kinase (MAPK) [100].

The octapeptide Ang II is not the only cleavage product obtained from the action of ACE2. Ang III, which is a C-terminal metabolite of Ang II, can also bind to the AT1 receptors, and is involved in the spinal nociceptive transmission [101]. Among the other products, there is the N-terminal metabolite Ang (1-7). It works by binding to the G-protein coupled receptor MAS which is expressed throughout the CNS and PNS including the DRG and spinal cord. Of note, Ang (1-7) may prevent the Ang II-induced nociceptive behavior via spinal MAS receptors (type 1) and the inhibition of p38 MAPK phosphorylation [102]. This heptapeptide can reduce proinflammatory cytokines such as TNF-α, IFN-γ, IL-1β, IL-6 while increasing the expression of the anti-inflammatory cytokine IL-10. In a mouse model of diabetic neuropathy, it was also demonstrated that Ang (1-7) may ameliorate the streptozotocin-induced diabetic neuropathic pain by acting on spinal MAS receptors and through the inhibition of p38 MAPK phosphorylation [103].

On these bases, the SARS-CoV-2 infection in the human spinal dorsal horn could upset the balance between two opposing systems: the ACE/Ang II/AT1 receptor axis and the ACE2/Ang (1–7)/MAS axis [104].

In this complex scenario, the AT2 receptor could play the role of protagonist/co-protagonist. It was proved that this receptor subtype is implicated in pain control [105]. Although the precise signaling pathway remains unclear, the receptor probably works as G-protein coupled receptor and, particularly in neurons, it provides the activation of the serine/threonine protein phosphatase 2A (PP2A). It leads to the generation of prostaglandin E2 from arachidonic acid by cyclooxygenase-1 (COX-1) and subsequent stimulation of the delayed rectifier K+ channel with hyperpolarization of plasma membranes. Other pathways concern the release of bradykinin and nitric oxide (NO). It was also proved that Ang II may provoke COX-2 induction [106]. All these processes are closed to the mechanisms of inflammation and nociception.

Previous in vitro (cultured human and rat DRG neurons) and animal studies showed that AT2 receptors were implicated in neurite outgrowth (after nerve injury), and thus in chronic pain and hypersensitivity associated with abnormal nerve sprouting [107]. In a rat model of neuropathic pain (chronic constriction injury of the sciatic nerve), an AT2 selective antagonist demonstrated important analgesic activity [108]. Furthermore, in a controlled clinical investigation, the AT2 receptor antagonist EMA401 ((S)-2-(diphenylacetyl)-1,2,3,4-tetrahydro-6-methoxy-5-(phenylmethoxy)-3-isoquinolinecarboxylic acid) was tested against post-herpetic neuropathic pain [109].

Considering these pieces of evidence, the alteration of nociception may not be necessarily produced by a virus/receptor (ACE2) within the CNS or PNS; it can be the effect of changes in the balance between the pathways of ACE2. It could be also hypothesized an upregulation of AT2 mediated (pro-nociceptive) mechanisms that are probably caused by excessive activation of the "classic" AT1 axis. Alternatively, or additionally, a functional imbalance between cytokine systems characterized by impairment of the Ang (1-7) pathway (anti-nociceptive) could occur. This could, at least in part, explain much of the painful manifestations in the absence of clear evidence of viral invasion into nerve tissue.

1.5.2 Long-Term Painful Clinical Manifestations

Patients who suffered from ARDS during their ICU stay are particularly prone to develop a post-discharge complex disorder featured by persistent fatigue, depression, weakness, and limited exercise tolerance which is defined as the distance walked in 6 min [110]. These problems have also been extensively described in SARS-survivors admitted to ICU [111].

The severity of the acute form of the infection is not an essential condition for the triggering of the post-COVID syndrome. It can also affect those who have not suffered from the most serious forms of the disease or those who have not been hospitalized. This syndrome, termed as long-COVID or post-COVID, has multiple clinical expressions and recognizes a multifactorial genesis. Painful manifestations such as myalgia, joint pain, headache, and others are encompassed within this set.

Among the pathogenic factors involved, there is the use of medications, such as systemic corticosteroids to manage the disease and multiorgan dysfunction, during the ICU stay. Additionally, a pivotal role is played by complex psycho-affective components including psychological effects of prolonged hospital admission, sleep, mood alterations, anxiety produced by separation, and isolation from family and friends. Factors strictly related to systemic inflammation like muscle atrophy due to immobility may contribute.

How many patients will need to be assisted because of chronic pain? Since the pandemic is still ongoing, it is difficult to have a precise estimate of the extent of the problem. It is also difficult to extrapolate data from epidemiological studies on SARS although SARS-CoV-2 is more contagious than SARS-CoV, the overall estimated case-fatality rate of COVID-19 is lower than the SARS. It must be considered that (i) about 5% of COVID-19 patients require ICU care; (ii) two-thirds of these may develop ARDS, and (iii) among ARDS COVID-19 cases, mortality estimate was 39% [112]. This is a very rough estimate in critically ill patients and the data could be very different considering all forms of the disease. On these premises, it is expected to have to assist several millions of COVID-19 survivors worldwide. Of these, an unspecified percentage will suffer from chronic non-specific pain. In a telephone follow-up of patients post-discharge ($n = 100$), compared to those affected by less severe forms of the disease, patients admitted to ICU showed a greater prevalence of non-specific pain (20–30% versus 10–20%), despite less affected by comorbidities [113].

Patients who experienced less severe forms (e.g., self-treated at home patients) may develop chronic pain and other post-COVID-19 clinical manifestations. In a follow-up study conducted 2 months after hospital discharge, the persistence of joint pain and chest pain was, respectively, 27.3% and 21.7% although the authors failed to report precise data on the illness severity [114]. Follow-up studies will be able to give us reliable data on the extent of the phenomenon. At the same time, assistance programs must be organized, in several clinical settings [115].

1.6 Ongoing Clinical Research

Given the enormous interest in COVID-19 neurotoxicity, many clinical studies have been planned on the subject. A schematic description of selected ongoing trials from several registries is shown in Table 1.2.

The "Norwegian Study of Nervous System Manifestations and Sequelae After COVID-19 (NeuroCovid)" (NCT04576351) is promoted by the Oslo University Hospital. It is a multi-center prospective observational clinical study of the

Table 1.2 Ongoing clinical research

Country	Design	Outcomes	Trial ID
Norway	Prospective Observational (multi-center)	Occurrence of neurological, Neuropsychological and psychiatric manifestations Clinical features and biomarkers	NCT04576351[a]
Swiss	Prospective observational	Influence of neurological complications on mortality and functional outcomes in ICU COVID-19 patients Imaging, EEG, and CSF. Histopathological findings	NCT04418609[a]
Germany	Prospective observational	Assessment of neuromuscular pathology Laboratory biomarkers and muscle ultrasound assessment	NCT04367350[a]
United States	Interventional	Rate of COVID-19 patients and underwent CAR-T therapy able to avoid death or MV	NCT04148430[a]
International	Prospective observational (multi-center)	Neurological, pulmonary, renal, liver function, and HR-QoL in post-ICU COVID-19 survivors	ACTRN 12620000799954p[b]

Abbreviations: *ICU* intensive care unit, *EEG* electroencephalography, *CSF* cerebrospinal fluid, *CAR-T* chimeric antigen receptor, *TMV* mechanical ventilation, *HR-QoL* health-related quality of life

[a]From the registry ClinicalTrials.gov

[b]From the Australian New Zealand Clinical Trials Registry (ANZCT) http://www.anzctr.org.au

occurrence of neurological, neuropsychological, and psychiatric manifestations and sequelae in patients with COVID-19. The study is aimed at identifying clinical features and biomarkers for both short- and long-term neurological treatment and rehabilitation. Blood samples for biomarker analyses, brain magnetic resonance imaging (MRI), clinical neurological, neurophysiological and neuropsychological assessments will be performed at 6 and 12 months after acute disease. The study began in September 2020 and is scheduled to end in December 2023, with the enrolment of 150 patients.

The impact of neurological complications on the course of the disease (e.g., mortality) and functional outcomes must be studied thoroughly. To this regard, the study titled "Neuro-COVID-19: Neurological Complications of COVID-19 (Neuro-COVID)" is a prospective observational cohort study aimed at evaluating the prevalence and severity of neurological symptoms among COVID-19 patients admitted to the ICU, as well as the influence of neurotoxicity on patients' outcomes (NCT04418609). The authors also planned to examine imaging, electroencephalography (EEG) data, and CSF analysis. They will also perform autopsies for analyzing pathological changes in the brain and histopathological findings, in those who die from the disease.

Another study is promoted by the Tübingen University Hospital, in Germany (NCT04367350). The researchers planned to perform a multimodal assessment of neuromuscular pathology associated with COVID-19-related ARDS. In particular, laboratory biomarkers (creatine kinase, troponin, urine myoglobin, and autoimmune antibodies) and muscle ultrasound assessment (Heckmatt score for the classification of muscle echogenicity) will be used.

Researchers from the Memorial Sloan Kettering Cancer Center (United States) are recruiting adult COVID-19 patients with a diagnosis of solid tumor or hematologic malignancies who underwent CAR-T. Their aim is to evaluate the effect of anakinra on both neurotoxicity and prevention of CRS secondary to CAR-T or COVID-19 (NCT04148430).

A long-term observation (up to 2 years post-ICU discharge) aimed at assessing neurological, pulmonary, renal, liver function, and health-related quality of life in COVID-19 survivors admitted to the ICU is performed through a multi-center international prospective study. In particular, cognitive impairment is assessed by the Montreal Cognitive Assessment and depression by the Patient-Health Questionnaire 9. The study was registered at the Australian New Zealand Clinical Trials Registry (ANZCT) (ACTRN12620000799954p).

1.7 Research Perspectives

Despite many papers have addressed the problem, multiple aspects related to COVID-19-induced neurotoxicity must be explained [116]. Research on pathophysiology must clear up many doubts (Table 1.3). For example, a crucial aspect is the correlation between the occurrence of neurological complications and the severity of the disease. While changes in taste and smell are common in non-severe COVID-19 forms and are not a predictor of severe disease, the same paradigm cannot be applied to the entire spectrum of neurological complications. The clinical experience suggests that the most severe neurological complications such as stroke and encephalopathy usually manifest in critically ill patients and are associated with significantly higher mortality.

Furthermore, the gender correlation and the role of age must be addressed. Interestingly, elderly patients were at an increased risk to suffer from myalgia, and fatigue, as compared with younger subjects who had a higher propensity to manifest symptoms related to sensorial disorders [117]. Furthermore, several investigations showed that young to middle-aged women are more prone to long-COVID [118].

Table 1.3 Main topics to be addressed on *neuro-COVID* research

Correlation between neurological complications and severity of the disease
The role of the gender, age, race factors
Genetic predisposition
The role of systemic conditions (e.g., hypoxemia, organ damage)
Precise mechanisms of neurotoxicity (e.g., the role of complement system)
Systemic effects of early neurological injury
Predictors of long-term complications
Tailored therapeutic approach

According to the "pregnancy compensation hypothesis," women of reproductive age have more reactive immune responses to a pathogen as their immune systems have evolved to support the heightened need for protection during pregnancy [119]. Another hypothesis assumes that the explanation can be traced back to autoimmune phenomena that are more evident in the female gender [120].

Is it possible that in some individuals there is a genetic predisposition to viral infection of nerve cells? Much could depend on the phenotypes of certain cytokines such as INFs that represent the protagonists of the innate immune barrier against viruses.

The pathophysiology must also clarify the dynamics of some neurological complications such as brain ischemia. It must be established whether sequelae are the effect of viral damage, or the consequence of an advanced state of the disease characterized by hypoxia and tissue hypoperfusion, combined or not with neuroinflammation. In critically ill COVID-19 patients, the occurrence of polyneuropathies could be explained by prolonged hospitalizations and neurotoxins production and configuring clinical pictures of critical illness polyneuropathy, or critical illness myopathy (especially in those requiring mechanical ventilation), rather than being labeled as specific COVID-19 clinical manifestations.

The study of neurological complications may also have other objectives. It may be possible, for example, to identify clinical-laboratory symptoms or signs suggestive of the severity of the disease, also concerning the development of the long-term sequelae. Furthermore, pathophysiology could offer important information to evaluate the possible consequences of early neurological damage. For instance, the rapid viral spread toward the CNS could explain the early respiratory complications which, in some cases, develop before that lung damage occurs [121].

The research must finally clarify the weight of the patient's general condition compared with the neurotropism of the virus, in the determinism of neurological complications. Factors such as hypoxia, multiorgan damage, could override the intrinsic ability of the virus to damage the CNS. As evidence of this, it has been found that elderly COVID-19 patients with hypertension, diabetes mellitus, and hyperlipidemia are at higher risk to develop ischemic stroke [122].

Regardless of whether the manifestations of neuro-COVID are produced by direct viral damage or they are secondary to the extent of the pathology and the inflammatory and immune-mediated systemic damage, it is appropriate to characterize the precise pathophysiology. It is also necessary to look for suggestive elements for brain damage. For instance, in the suspicion of an encephalitic-like involvement, it could be suggested to calculate the albumin and IgG indices to determine BBB permeability.

Since pathophysiological data indicate that elderly patients are exposed to an acceleration of cognitive decline following COVID-19, clinical research, but also preclinical investigations, must pay attention to potential strategies aimed at the prevention of post-infection neurocognitive damages. In this context, several anti-aging therapeutics such as sirtuins, quercetin, and fisetin can be tested. Another important argument to be addressed is the role of nutrition, especially for ICU patients. Vitamins deficiency, for example, can be associated with musculoskeletal pain [123]. Moreover, as a retrospective analysis showed, the problem seems to affect not only ICU patients [124]. Epidemiological studies conducted on different populations are needed to provide more detailed data.

From preclinical and translational research, a detailed understanding of the cascade of events leading to nervous tissue damage is expected. To meet this fundamental objective, it is necessary:

(a) To design in vitro, in vivo, and in silico ad hoc models that can recapitulate the physiological effects of SARS-CoV-2 infection. In particular, studies are needed to define how SARS-CoV-2 gains access to the brain, dissect mechanisms of the neuroimmune activation, and illustrate the distribution of the virus in the brain.
(b) To characterize the pathogenetic processes that are triggered by the action of the virus and the host's response. For example, multiple features of severe SARS-CoV-2 infection suggest that complement activation plays a pivotal role in the pathogenesis of COVID-19, particularly during exaggerated immune responses [125]. Other interesting elements in the cascade, such as the potential immune-mediated disruption of the autonomic nervous system, need to be better characterized [126].
(c) To develop a therapy approach tailored to different steps in the cascade. In this regard, a very interesting randomized, parallel, multi-center phase I/II clinical trial is ongoing (NCT04324996). Because natural killer (NK) cells are the major cells of the natural immune system with a paramount role against virus infection, researchers are testing an activating receptor of these cells (NKG2D) to enhance the clearing of SARS-CoV-2 infected cells. The study provides the development of NK cells modified by CAR technology. In brief, the NKG2D-ACE2 CAR-NK cells secreting an IL-15 "superagonist" capable of CRS prevention and granulocyte-macrophage colony-stimulating factor (GM-CSF) neutralizing. This strategy could be also effective for preventing neurotoxicity as CAR-T-related neurotoxicity can be counteracted through GM-CSF neutralization [127].

Although clinical research is usually inspired by data obtained from preclinical research, building a research design starting from clinical data is often a difficult task of translational research. In this context, the influence of treatment regimens of neurological complications could help to clarify doubts about the pathogenesis of neuro-COVID.

Important findings could also be transferred from the imaging research. In a study carried out on patients with COVID-19 admitted to the ICU with neurologic signs, brain MRI showed leptomeningeal enhancement [128]. In another study focused on the topic, it was found that the MRI findings in COVID-19 ICU patients consisted of leptomeningeal enhancement but also cortical signal intensity abnormalities on fluid-attenuated inversion recovery images, and cortical diffusion restriction. These non-specific imaging patterns suggest that neurological changes need to be very carefully interpreted as they can be also detected in infectious or autoimmune encephalitis, seizure, hypoglycemia, and hypoxia. Doubtless, as the authors stated, further research is needed to establish imaging patterns suggestive for neurotropism of COVID-19 [129].

The most important data expected from the research is to provide evidence of the actual presence of the virus within the brain and CSF. If failing to detect the virus is only a matter of "false negative" results, more useful biomarkers for infection of the CNS such as PCR and antibodies against SARS-CoV-2 in CSF must be necessarily developed. Previously, the RNA sequence of the HCoV OC43 was detected in brain biopsies in immunosuppressed children with encephalitis [91], and SARS-CoV was isolated in brain tissue of patients who died of SARS [130]. Nevertheless, to date, the scientific evidence on SARS-CoV-2 can only refer to sporadic reports and, although conducted on a limited number of patients, ad hoc investigations have failed to detect SARS-CoV-2 in the CSF [131].

About clinical settings, it would be interesting to evaluate the extent of neurotoxicity in cancer patients. The translational research offers important data. For instance, since TMPRSS2 expression is highly increased in cancers cells and it is also directly correlated with the degree of cancer pain [132], in this vulnerable population the problem of COVID-pain could represent a great concern.

Finally, if the virus is really capable of infecting nerve cells, what could be the effect of this viral stay on the long-term sequelae? Given the clinical, social, and healthcare impact this is a question of enormous importance.

1.8 Conclusions

Several coronaviruses, including some HCoVs are naturally neuroinvasive, neurotropic, and neurovirulent and can potentially disseminate within the CNS. Could the same argument also apply to SARS-CoV-2? To date, it is not possible to answer this question with certainty.

Therefore, it is necessary to leverage on what we currently know about the matter (Table 1.4).

Since the ACE2 receptor is expressed in neurons and glial cells, and SARS-CoV-2 binds to the ACE2 with a higher affinity than that of SARS-CoV, the logical inference is that the former HCoV could be more capable of infecting and damaging the CNS than SARS-CoV. Nevertheless, there is no direct evidence for

Table 1.4 What do we know on SARS-CoV-2 neurotoxicity

The host receptor, ACE2, is expressed in neurons and glial cells
There are no direct evidence for a SARS-CoV-2-caused CNS damage
There are no proofs of a fulminant virus-induced encephalitis
Although the precise route is still debated, the virus is able to gain access to the brain
Apart from ACE2, other factors (co-receptors) can be involved
The neuropathological alterations are most likely to be immune mediated

SARS-CoV-2-caused CNS damage. Additionally, although the virus has potential neurological effects, and clinical practice is progressively delineating the picture of the COVID-19-associated neurotoxicity or simply neuro-COVID, the mechanisms of neural damage should be better investigated.

Another big unknown in neurotoxicity is whether the virus produces a direct attack or the damage to the nervous tissue is produced by an indirect (inflammatory and immune-mediated) insult. The neurotoxicity, indeed, can be the effect of aberrant activation of the immune system. Probably, multiple mechanisms occur, even in combination.

There are two anatomical routes for a virus to enter the CNS: (i) a neural pathway and (ii) a body fluid such as blood, lymph, and CSF. Concerning SARS-CoV-2, the neural pathway may follow mainly the olfactory tract for invading, in turn, the CNS. On the other hand, the body fluid way is primarily performed through the hematogenous route.

Regardless of the pathway used, the viruses exert their neurotropism through binding to host receptors, especially ACE2. Since neurons and glial cells express ACE-2 receptors, they are both potential targets. Nevertheless, other factors are necessarily involved in the SARS-CoV-2 neurotropism. Numerous studies have been conducted on the subject. Many other scientific achievements must be added to them. Pieces of evidence come from studies on other HCoVs, or are extrapolated from other research fields. Translational research, in fact, has made it possible to acquire a lot of useful information for trying to untangle this tangled skein.

The cytokine storm is a real dilemma for scientists and clinicians. Since it is an atomic explosion triggered inside a nuclear reactor, it appears to be capable of producing all sorts of damage. In COVID-19, lung lesions are a typical example of this explosion and neurological damage has impeccable logic. These immune-mediated neurological injuries can manifest either during or after the viral infection.

The ultimate of the research on underlined mechanisms of SARS-CoV-2-induced neurotoxicity remains the need to implement appropriate prophylactic and therapeutic measures. The concept is valid not only for acute complications such as headache, and sensory alterations, but also and above all for addressing the paramount issue of the potential long-term neurological and psychological sequelae. This latter aspect creates many concerns. Even after the resolution of the clinical picture of the disease, patients can develop memory loss, confusion, and other forms of neurocognitive impairment. The genesis seems to be multifactorial, with the combination of viral damage, effects of hypoxia, consequences of more or less invasive therapies, effects of isolation of critically ill patients. Determining the factors involved and the weight of each appears to be a challenge that will keep researchers busy for a long time after the pandemic is resolved. It is reasonable to assume that only studies with long-term follow-up and evidence-based medicine data will provide us with adequate answers. In the meantime, we need to intensify preclinical investigations, enhance translational research, and collect as much as clinical data possible.

References

1. Gupta A, Madhavan MV, Sehgal K, et al. Extrapulmonary manifestations of COVID-19. Nat Med. 2020;26:1017–32.
2. Al-Samkari H, Karp Leaf RS, Dzik WH, et al. COVID-19 and coagulation: bleeding and thrombotic manifestations of SARS-CoV-2 infection. Blood. 2020;136(4):489–500. https://doi.org/10.1182/blood.2020006520.
3. Magadum A, Kishore R. Cardiovascular Manifestations of COVID-19 Infection. Cell. 2020;9(11):2508. https://doi.org/10.3390/cells9112508.
4. Asgharpour M, Zare E, Mubarak M, Alirezaei A. COVID-19 and kidney disease: update on epidemiology, clinical manifestations, pathophysiology and management. J Coll Physicians Surg Pak. 2020;30(6):19–25. https://doi.org/10.29271/jcpsp.2020.Supp1.S19.
5. Patel KP, Patel PA, Vunnam RR, Hewlett AT, Jain R, Jing R, Vunnam SR. Gastrointestinal, hepatobiliary, and pancreatic manifestations of COVID-19. J Clin Virol. 2020;128:104386. https://doi.org/10.1016/j.jcv.2020.104386.
6. Marazuela M, Giustina A, Puig-Domingo M. Endocrine and metabolic aspects of the COVID-19 pandemic. Rev Endocr Metab Disord. 2020;21(4):495–507. https://doi.org/10.1007/s11154-020-09569-2. Erratum in: Rev Endocr Metab Disord. 2021 Jan 6
7. Wu P, Duan F, Luo C, Liu Q, Qu X, Liang L, Wu K. Characteristics of ocular findings of patients with coronavirus disease 2019 (COVID-19) in Hubei Province, China. JAMA Ophthalmol. 2020;138(5):575–8. https://doi.org/10.1001/jamaophthalmol.2020.1291.
8. Gianotti R, Veraldi S, Recalcati S, et al. Cutaneous clinico-pathological findings in three COVID-19-positive patients observed in the metropolitan area of Milan, Italy. Acta Derm Venereol. 2020,100(8):adv00124. https://doi.org/10.2340/00015555-3490.
9. Niazkar HR, Zibaee B, Nasimi A, Bahri N. The neurological manifestations of COVID-19: a review article. Neurol Sci. 2020;41(7):1667–71. https://doi.org/10.1007/s10072-020-04486-3.
10. Khatoon F, Prasad K, Kumar V. Neurological manifestations of COVID-19: available evidences and a new paradigm. J Neurovirol. 2020;26(5):619–30. https://doi.org/10.1007/s13365-020-00895-4.
11. Gu J, Gong E, Zhang B, et al. Multiple organ infection and the pathogenesis of SARS. J Exp Med. 2005;202(3):415–24.
12. Desforges M, Le Coupanec A, Stodola JK, Meessen-Pinard M, Talbot PJ. Human coronaviruses: viral and cellular factors involved in neuroinvasiveness and neuropathogenesis. Virus Res. 2014;194:145–58.
13. Talbot PJ, Ekandé S, Cashman NR, Mounir S, Stewart JN. Neurotropism of human coronavirus 229E. Adv Exp Med Biol. 1993;342:339–46.
14. Mentis AA, Dardiotis E, Grigoriadis N, Petinaki E, Hadjigeorgiou GM. Viruses and endogenous retroviruses in multiple sclerosis: from correlation to causation. Acta Neurol Scand. 2017;136(6):606–16.
15. Greig AS, Mitchell D, Corner AH, Bannister GL, Meads EB, Julian RJ. A hemagglutinating virus producing encephalomyelitis in baby pigs. Can J Comp Med Vet Sci. 1962;26(3):49–56.
16. Burks JS, DeVald BL, Jankovsky LD, Gerdes JC. Two coronaviruses isolated from central nervous system tissue of two multiple sclerosis patients. Science. 1980;209(4459):933–4.
17. Lane TE, Hosking MP. The pathogenesis of murine coronavirus infection of the central nervous system. Crit Rev Immunol. 2010;30:119–30.
18. Perrone F, Piccirillo MC, Ascierto PA, TOCIVID-19 Investigators, Italy, et al. Tocilizumab for patients with COVID-19 pneumonia. The single-arm TOCIVID-19 prospective trial. J Transl Med. 2020;18(1):405. https://doi.org/10.1186/s12967-020-02573-9.
19. Bimonte S, Crispo A, Amore A, Celentano E, Cuomo A, Cascella M. Potential antiviral drugs for SARS-Cov-2 treatment: preclinical findings and ongoing clinical research. In Vivo. 2020;34(Suppl. 3):1597–602. https://doi.org/10.21873/invivo.11949.
20. Buonaguro FM, Botti G, Ascierto PA, the INT-Pascale COVID-19 Crisis Unit, et al. The clinical and translational research activities at the INT—IRCCS "Fondazione Pascale" cancer

center (Naples, Italy) during the COVID-19 pandemic. Infect Agent Cancer. 2020;15(1):69. https://doi.org/10.1186/s13027-020-00330-7.
21. Cascella M, Mauro I, De Blasio E, et al. Rapid and impressive response to a combined treatment with single-dose tocilizumab and NIV in a patient with COVID-19 pneumonia/ARDS. Medicina (Kaunas). 2020;56(8):377. https://doi.org/10.3390/medicina56080377.
22. Giacomelli A, Pezzati L, Conti F, Bernacchia D, Siano M. Oreni L (2020) Self-reported olfactory and taste disorders in SARS-CoV-2 patients: a cross-sectional study. Clin Infect Dis. 2020; https://doi.org/10.1093/cid/ciaa330.
23. Li LQ, Huang T, Wang YQ, et al. COVID-19 patients' clinical characteristics, discharge rate, and fatality rate of meta-analysis. J Med Virol. 2020;92(6):577–83. https://doi.org/10.1002/jmv.25757.
24. Lechien JR, Chiesa-Estomba CM, De Siati DR, et al. Olfactory and gustatory dysfunctions as a clinical presentation of mild-to-moderate forms of the coronavirus disease (COVID-19): a multicenter European study. Eur Arch Otorhinolaryngol. 2020;277:1–11. https://doi.org/10.1007/s00405-020-05965-1.
25. Zhu J, Zhong Z, Ji P, Pang J, Zhang J, Zhao C. Clinicopathological characteristics of 8697 patients with COVID-19 in China: a meta-analysis. Fam Med Community Health. 2020;8(2):e000406. https://doi.org/10.1136/fmch-2020-000406.
26. Paliwal VK, Garg RK, Gupta A, Tejan N. Neuromuscular presentations in patients with COVID-19. Neurol Sci. 2020;41(11):3039–56.
27. Vittori A, Lerman J, Cascella M, et al. COVID-19 Pandemic acute respiratory distress syndrome survivors: pain after the storm? Anesth Analg. 2020;131(1):117–9. https://doi.org/10.1213/ANE.0000000000004914.
28. Finsterer J, Stollberger C. Update on the neurology of COVID-19. J Med Virol. 2020;92(11):2316–8.
29. Asadi-Pooya AA, Simani L. Central nervous system manifestations of COVID-19: a systematic review. J Neurol Sci. 2020;413:116832. https://doi.org/10.1016/j.jns.2020.116832.
30. Whittaker A, Anson M, Harky A. Neurological Manifestations of COVID-19: a systematic review and current update. Acta Neurol Scand. 2020;142(1):14–22.
31. To KF, Tong JH, Chan PK, et al. Tissue and cellular tropism of the coronavirus associated with severe acute respiratory syndrome: an in-situ hybridization study of fatal cases. J Pathol. 2004;202(2):157–63.
32. Puelles VG, Lütgehetmann M, Lindenmeyer MT, et al. Multiorgan and renal tropism of SARS-CoV-2. N Engl J Med. 2020;383(6):590–2. https://doi.org/10.1056/NEJMc2011400.
33. Schaller T, Hirschbuhl K, Burkhardt K. Postmortem examination of patients with COVID-19. JAMA. 2020;2020:323.
34. Matschke J, Lütgehetmann M, Hagel C, et al. Neuropathology of patients with COVID-19 in Germany: a post-mortem case series. Lancet Neurol. 2020;19(11):919–29. https://doi.org/10.1016/S1474-4422(20)30308-2.
35. Goranci-Buzhala G, Mariappan A, et al. Rapid and efficient invasion assay of glioblastoma in human brain organoids. Cell Rep. 2020;31:107738.
36. Ramani A, Müller L, Ostermann PN, et al (2020) SARS-CoV-2 targets neurons of 3D human brain organoids. EMBO J 39(20):e106230. https://doi.org/10.15252/embj.2020106230.
37. Moriguchi T, Harii N, Goto J, et al. A first case of meningitis/encephalitis associated with SARS-Coronavirus-2. Int J Infect Dis. 2020;94:55–8.
38. Alexopoulos H, Magira E, Bitzogli K, et al. Anti-SARS-CoV-2 antibodies in the CSF, blood-brain barrier dysfunction, and neurological outcome: studies in 8 stuporous and comatose patients. Neurol Neuroimmunol Neuroinflamm. 2020;7(6):e893. https://doi.org/10.1212/NXI.0000000000000893.
39. Kremer S, Lersy F, de Sèze J, et al. Brain MRI findings in severe COVID-19: a retrospective observational study. Radiology. 2020;297(2):E242–51. https://doi.org/10.1148/radiol.2020202222.

40. Lu Y, Li X, Geng D, et al. Cerebral micro-structural changes in COVID-19 patients—an MRI-based 3-month follow-up study. EClinicalMedicine. 2020;25:100484. https://doi.org/10.1016/j.eclinm.2020.100484.
41. Netland J, Meyerholz DK, Moore S, Cassell M, Perlman S. Severe acute respiratory syndrome coronavirus infection causes neuronal death in the absence of encephalitis in mice transgenic for human ACE2. J Virol. 2008;82(15):7264–75.
42. Lau KK, Yu WC, Chu CM, Lau ST, Sheng B, Yuen KY. Possible central nervous system infection by SARS coronavirus. Emerg Infect Dis. 2004;10(2):342–4.
43. Xu J, Zhong S, Liu J, et al. Detection of severe acute respiratory syndrome coronavirus in the brain: potential role of the chemokine mig in pathogenesis. Clin Infect Dis. 2005;41(8):1089–96.
44. Santos RAS, Sampaio WO, Alzamora AC, et al. The ACE2/Angiotensin-(1-7)/MAS Axis of the renin-angiotensin system: Focus on angiotensin-(1-7). Physiol Rev. 2018;98:505–53. https://doi.org/10.1152/physrev.00023.2016.
45. Alon R, Sportiello M, Kozlovski S, et al. Leukocyte trafficking to the lungs and beyond: lessons from influenza for COVID-19. Nat Rev Immunol. 2021;21:49–64.
46. Steckelings UM, Unger T. Angiotensin II type 2 receptor agonists—where should they be applied? Expert Opin Investig Drugs. 2012;21(6):763–6.
47. Li Y, Zhang Z, Yang L, et al. The MERS-CoV receptor DPP4 as a candidate binding target of the SARS-CoV-2 Spike. iScience. 2020;23(6):101160. https://doi.org/10.1016/j.isci.2020.101160.
48. Wölfel R, Corman VM, Guggemos W, et al. Virological assessment of hospitalized patients with COVID-2019. Nature. 2020;581(7809):465–9. https://doi.org/10.1038/s41586-020-2196-x.
49. Coutard B, Valle C, de Lamballerie X, et al. The spike glycoprotein of the new coronavirus 2019-nCoV contains a furin-like cleavage site absent in CoV of the same clade. Antivir Res. 2020;176:104742. https://doi.org/10.1016/j.antiviral.2020.104742pmid:32057769.
50. Tse LV, Hamilton AM, Friling T, Whittaker GR. A novel activation mechanism of avian influenza virus H9N2 by furin. J Virol. 2014;88:1673 83. https://doi.org/10.1128/JVI.02648-13pmid:24257604.
51. Li MY, Li L, Zhang Y, Wang XS. Expression of the SARS-CoV-2 cell receptor gene ACE2 in a wide variety of human tissues. Infect Dis Poverty. 2020;9(1):45.
52. Matsuyama S, Nao N, Shirato K, et al. Enhanced isolation of SARS-CoV-2 by TMPRSS2-expressing cells. Proc Natl Acad Sci U S A. 2020;117(13):7001–3.
53. Gomes CP, Fernandes DE, Casimiro F, et al. Cathepsin L in COVID-19: from pharmacological evidences to genetics. Front Cell Infect Microbiol. 2020;10:589505. https://doi.org/10.3389/fcimb.2020.589505.
54. Bullen CK, Hogberg HT, Bahadirli-Talbott A, et al. Infectability of human BrainSphere neurons suggests neurotropism of SARS-CoV-2. ALTEX. 2020;37(4):665–71. https://doi.org/10.14573/altex.2006111.
55. Qiao J, Li W, Bao J, et al. The expression of SARS-CoV-2 receptor ACE2 and CD147, and protease TMPRSS2 in human and mouse brain cells and mouse brain tissues. Biochem Biophys Res Commun. 2020;533(4):867–71.
56. Curtin KD, Wyman RJ, Meinertzhagen IA. Basigin/EMMPRIN/CD147 mediates neuron-glia interactions in the optic lamina of Drosophila. Glia. 2007;55(15):1542–53. https://doi.org/10.1002/glia.20568.
57. Cascella M, Bimonte S, Barbieri A, et al. Dissecting the potential roles of Nigella sativa and its constituent thymoquinone on the prevention and on the progression of Alzheimer's disease. Front Aging Neurosci. 2018;10:16. https://doi.org/10.3389/fnagi.2018.00016.
58. Cascella M, Bimonte S, Muzio MR, Schiavone V, Cuomo A. The efficacy of Epigallocatechin-3-gallate (green tea) in the treatment of Alzheimer's disease: an overview of pre-clinical studies and translational perspectives in clinical practice. Infect Agent Cancer. 2017;12:36. https://doi.org/10.1186/s13027-017-0145-6.

59. Lu M, Wu J, Hao ZW, et al. Basolateral CD147 induces hepatocyte polarity loss by E-cadherin ubiquitination and degradation in hepatocellular carcinoma progress. Hepatology. 2018;1:317–32.
60. Wang K, Chen W, Zhang Z, et al. CD147-spike protein is a novel route for SARS-CoV-2 infection to host cells. Signal Transduct Target Ther. 2020;5(1):283. https://doi.org/10.1038/s41392-020-00426-x.
61. Agrawal SM, Silva C, Tourtellotte WW, Yong VW. EMMPRIN: a novel regulator of leukocyte transmigration into the CNS in multiple sclerosis and experimental autoimmune encephalomyelitis. J Neurosci. 2011;31(2):669–77. https://doi.org/10.1523/JNEUROSCI.3659-10.2011.
62. Cantuti-Castelvetri L, Ojha R, Pedro LD, et al. Neuropilin-1 facilitates SARS-CoV-2 cell entry and infectivity. Science. 2020;6518:856–60.
63. Xiao F, Tang M, Zheng X, Liu Y, Li X, Shan H. Evidence for Gastrointestinal Infection of SARS-CoV-2. Gastroenterology. 2020;158(6):1831–3. e3
64. Deng W, Bao L, Gao H, et al. Ocular conjunctival inoculation of SARS-CoV-2 can cause mild COVID-19 in rhesus macaques. Nat Commun. 2020;11(1):4400. https://doi.org/10.1038/s41467-020-18149-6.
65. Paniz-Mondolfi A, Bryce C, Grimes Z, et al. Central nervous system involvement by severe acute respiratory syndrome coronavirus-2 (SARS-CoV-2). J Med Virol. 2020;92(7):699–702.
66. Rhea EM, Logsdon AF, Hansen KM, et al. The S1 protein of SARS-CoV-2 crosses the blood–brain barrier in mice. Nat Neurosci. 2020; https://doi.org/10.1038/s41593-020-00771-8.
67. van Riel D, Verdijk R, Kuiken T. The olfactory nerve: a shortcut for influenza and other viral diseases into the central nervous system. J Pathol. 2015;235(2):277–87.
68. Hornuss D, Lange B, Schröter N, Rieg S, Kern WV, Wagner D. Anosmia in COVID-19 patients. Clin Microbiol Infect. 2020;26(10):1426–7.
69. Rodrigues Prestes TR, Rocha NP, Miranda AS, Teixeira AL, Simoes-e-Silva AC. The anti-inflammatory potential of ACE2/angiotensin-(1-7)/mas receptor axis: evidence from basic and clinical research. Curr Drug Targets. 2017;18:1301–13.
70. Perlman S, Jacobsen G, Afifi A. Spread of a neurotropic murine coronavirus into the CNS via the trigeminal and olfactory nerves. Virology. 1989;170(2):556–60.
71. Bohmwald K, Gálvez NMS, Ríos M, Kalergis AM. Neurologic alterations due to respiratory virus infections. Front Cell Neurosci. 2018;12:386.
72. Sun XF, Zhang X, Chen XH, et al. The infection evidence of SARS-COV-2 in ocular surface: a single-center cross-sectional study. medRxiv. 2020; https://doi.org/10.1101/2020.02.26.20027938.
73. Dubé M, Le Coupanec A, Wong A, Rini JM, Desforges M, Talbot PJ. Axonal transport enables neuron-to-neuron propagation of human coronavirus OC43. J Virol. 2018;92(17):e00404–18.
74. Li YC, Bai WZ, Hirano N, Hayashida T, Hashikawa T. Coronavirus infection of rat dorsal root ganglia: ultrastructural characterization of viral replication, transfer, and the early response of satellite cells. Virus Res. 2012;163(2):628–35.
75. Lima M, Siokas V, Aloizou AM, et al. Unraveling the possible routes of SARS-COV-2 invasion into the central nervous system. Curr Treat Options Neurol. 2020;22(11):37. https://doi.org/10.1007/s11940-020-00647-z.
76. Ratajczak J, Wysoczynski M, Hayek F, Janowska-Wieczorek A, Ratajczak MZ. Membrane-derived microvesicles: Important and underappreciated mediators of cell-to-cell communication. Leukemia. 2006;20:1487–95.
77. Varga Z, Flammer AJ, Steiger P, Haberecker M, et al. Endothelial cell infection and endotheliitis in COVID-19. Lancet. 2020;395(10234):1417–8. https://doi.org/10.1016/S0140-6736(20)30937-5.
78. Lau SK-P, Lau CCY, Chan K-H, et al. Delayed induction of proinflammatory cytokines and suppression of innate antiviral response by the Novel Middle East respiratory syndrome coronavirus: implications for pathogenesis and treatment. J Gen Virol. 2013;94:2679–90.
79. Conti P, Ronconi G, Caraffa A, et al. Induction of pro-inflammatory cytokines (IL-1 and IL-6) and lung inflammation by Coronavirus-19 (COVI-19 or SARS-CoV-2): anti-inflammatory strategies. J Biol Regul Homeost Agents. 2020;34(2):327–31.

80. Adinolfi E, Giuliani AL, De Marchi E, Pegoraro A, Orioli E, Di Virgilio F. The P2X7 receptor: a main player in inflammation. Biochem Pharmacol. 2018;151:234–44.
81. Ribeiro DE, Oliveira-Giacomelli Á, Glaser T, et al. Hyperactivation of P2X7 receptors as a culprit of COVID-19 neuropathology. Mol Psychiatr. 2020; https://doi.org/10.1038/s41380-020-00965-3.
82. Li Y, Fu L, Gonzales DM, Lavi E. Coronavirus correlates with the ability of the virus to induce proinflammatory cytokine signals from astrocytes and microglia. J Virol. 2004;78:3398–406.
83. Wiersinga WJ, Rhodes A, Cheng AC, Peacock SJ, Prescott HC. Pathophysiology, transmission, diagnosis, and treatment of coronavirus disease 2019 (COVID-19): a review. JAMA. 2020;324(8):782–93.
84. Brudno JN, Kochenderfer JN. Recent advances in CAR T-cell toxicity: mechanisms, manifestations and management. Blood Rev. 2019:45–55. https://doi.org/10.1016/j.blre.2018.11.002.
85. Gust J, Hay KA, Hanafi LA, et al. Endothelial activation and blood-brain barrier disruption in neurotoxicity after adoptive immunotherapy with CD19 CAR-T cells. Cancer Discov. 2017;7(12):1404–19.
86. Cascella M, Muzio MR, Bimonte S, Cuomo A, Jakobsson JG. Postoperative delirium and postoperative cognitive dysfunction: updates in pathophysiology, potential translational approaches to clinical practice and further research perspectives. Minerva Anestesiol. 2018;84(2):246–60. https://doi.org/10.23736/S0375-9393.17.12146-2.
87. Cascella M, Bimonte S. The role of general anesthetics and the mechanisms of hippocampal and extra-hippocampal dysfunctions in the genesis of postoperative cognitive dysfunction. Neural Regen Res. 2017;12(11):1780–5. https://doi.org/10.4103/1673-5374.219032.
88. Cascella M, Di Napoli R, Carbone D, Cuomo GF, Bimonte S, Muzio MR. Chemotherapy-related cognitive impairment: mechanisms, clinical features and research perspectives. Recenti Prog Med. 2018;109(11):523–30. https://doi.org/10.1701/3031.30289.
89. Ferro JM, Caeiro L, Figueira ML. Neuropsychiatric sequelae of stroke. Nat Rev Neurol. 2016;12:269–80.
90. Roe K, Kumar M, Lum S, Orillo B, Nerurkar VR, Verma S. West Nile virus-induced disruption of the blood-brain barrier in mice is characterized by the degradation of the junctional complex proteins and increase in multiple matrix metalloproteinases. J Gen Virol. 2012;93(Pt 6):1193–203.
91. Unni SK, Růžek D, Chhatbar C, Mishra R, Johri MK, Singh SK. Japanese encephalitis virus: from genome to infectome. Microbes Infect. 2011;13:312–21.
92. Shinu P, Morsy MA, Deb PK, et al. SARS CoV-2 Organotropism Associated Pathogenic Relationship of Gut-Brain Axis and Illness. Front Mol Biosci. 2020;7:606779. https://doi.org/10.3389/fmolb.2020.606779.
93. Xiao H, Zhang Y, Kong D, Li S, Yang N. The effects of social support on sleep quality of medical staff treating patients with coronavirus disease 2019 (COVID-19) in January and February 2020 in China. Med Sci Monit. 2020;26:e923549. https://doi.org/10.12659/MSM.923921.
94. Hascup ER, Hascup KN. Does SARS-CoV-2 infection cause chronic neurological complications? Geroscience. 2020;42(4):1083–7. https://doi.org/10.1007/s11357-020-00207-y.
95. Diniz BS, Reynolds CF 3rd, Begley A, et al. Brain-derived neurotrophic factor levels in late-life depression and comorbid mild cognitive impairment: a longitudinal study. J Psychiatr Res. 2014;49:96–101.
96. Baig AM. Deleterious outcomes in long-hauler COVID-19: the effects of SARS-CoV-2 on the CNS in chronic COVID syndrome. ACS Chem Neurosci. 2020;11(24):4017–20. https://doi.org/10.1021/acschemneuro.0c00725.
97. Doykov I, Hällqvist J, Gilmour KC, et al. The long tail of Covid-19′ - The detection of a prolonged inflammatory response after a SARS-CoV-2 infection in asymptomatic and mildly affected patients. F1000Res. 2020;9:1349. https://doi.org/10.12688/f1000research.27287.2.

98. Cascella M, Del Gaudio A, Vittori A, Bimonte S, Del Prete P, Forte CA, Cuomo A, De Blasio E. COVID-Pain: Acute and Late-Onset Painful Clinical Manifestations in COVID-19 - Molecular Mechanisms and Research Perspectives. J Pain Res. 2021;14:2403–12. https://doi.org/10.2147/JPR.S313978.
99. Nemoto W, Yamagata R, Nakagawasai O, et al. Effect of spinal angiotensin-converting enzyme 2 activation on the formalin-induced nociceptive response in mice. Eur J Pharmacol. 2020;872:172950. https://doi.org/10.1016/j.ejphar.2020.172950.
100. Nemoto W, Nakagawasai O, Yaoita F, et al. Angiotensin II produces nociceptive behavior through spinal AT1 receptor-mediated p38 mitogen-activated protein kinase activation in mice. Mol Pain. 2013;9:38. https://doi.org/10.1186/1744-8069-9-38.
101. Nemoto W, Ogata Y, Nakagawasai O, Yaoita F, Tadano T, Tan-No K. Involvement of p38 MAPK activation mediated through AT1 receptors on spinal astrocytes and neurons in angiotensin II- and III-induced nociceptive behavior in mice. Neuropharmacology. 2015;99:221–31.
102. Yamagata R, Nemoto W, Nakagawasai O, Takahashi K, Tan-No K. Downregulation of spinal angiotensin converting enzyme 2 is involved in neuropathic pain associated with type 2 diabetes mellitus in mice. Biochem Pharmacol. 2020;174:113825. https://doi.org/10.1016/j.bcp.2020.113825.
103. Ogata Y, Nemoto W, Yamagata R, et al. Anti-hypersensitive effect of angiotensin (1-7) on streptozotocin-induced diabetic neuropathic pain in mice. Eur J Pain. 2019;23(4):739–49.
104. Su S, Cui H, Wang T, Shen X, Ma C. Pain: a potential new label of COVID-19. Brain Behav Immun. 2020;87:159–60. https://doi.org/10.1016/j.bbi.2020.05.025.
105. Danser AH, Anand P. The angiotensin II type 2 receptor for pain control. Cell. 2014;157(7):1504–6.
106. Soda K, Nakada Y, Iwanari H. Hamakubo T (2020) AT2 receptor interacting protein 1 (ATIP1) mediates COX-2 induction by an AT2 receptor agonist in endothelial cells. Biochem Biophys Rep. 2020;24:100850. https://doi.org/10.1016/j.bbrep.2020.100850.
107. Anand U, Facer P, Yiangou Y, et al. Angiotensin II type 2 receptor (AT2 R) localization and antagonist-mediated inhibition of capsaicin responses and neurite outgrowth in human and rat sensory neurons. Eur J Pain. 2013;17(7):1012–26.
108. Smith MT, Woodruff TM, Wyse BD, Muralidharan A, Walther T. A small molecule angiotensin II type 2 receptor (AT2R) antagonist produces analgesia in a rat model of neuropathic pain by inhibition of p38 mitogen-activated protein kinase (MAPK) and p44/p42 MAPK activation in the dorsal root ganglia. Pain Med. 2013;14(10):1557–68.
109. Rice ASC, Dworkin RH, McCarthy TD, et al. EMA401, an orally administered highly selective angiotensin II type 2 receptor antagonist, as a novel treatment for postherpetic neuralgia: a randomised, double-blind, placebo-controlled phase 2 clinical trial. Lancet. 2014;383:1637–47.
110. Bein T, Weber-Carstens S, Apfelbacher C. Long-term out-come after the acute respiratory distress syndrome: different from general critical illness? Curr Opin Crit Care. 2018;24:35–40.
111. Moldofsky H, Patcai J. Chronic widespread musculoskeletal pain, fatigue, depression and disordered sleep in chronic post-SARS syndrome; a case-controlled study. BMC Neurol. 2011;11:37.
112. Hasan SS, Capstick T, Ahmed R, et al. Mortality in COVID-19 patients with acute respiratory distress syndrome and corticosteroids use: a systematic review and meta-analysis. Expert Rev Respir Med. 2020;14(11):1149–63.
113. Halpin SJ, McIvor C, Whyatt G, et al. Postdischarge symptoms and rehabilitation needs in survivors of COVID-19 infection: a cross-sectional evaluation. J Med Virol. 2021;93(2):1013–22.
114. Carfì A, Bernabei R, Landi F, Gemelli Against COVID-19 Post-Acute Care Study Group. Persistent symptoms in patients after acute COVID-19. JAMA. 2020;324(6):603–5.
115. Crispo A, Montagnese C, Perri F, et al. COVID-19 Emergency and post-emergency in Italian cancer patients: how can patients be assisted? Front Oncol. 2020;10:1571. https://doi.org/10.3389/fonc.2020.01571.

116. Huang J, Zheng M, Tang X, Chen Y, Tong A, Zhou L. Potential of SARS-CoV-2 to cause CNS infection: biologic fundamental and clinical experience. Front Neurol. 2020;11:659. https://doi.org/10.3389/fneur.2020.00659.
117. Lechien JR, Chiesa-Estomba CM, Place S, et al. Clinical and epidemiological characteristics of 1420 European patients with mild-to-moderate coronavirus disease 2019. J Intern Med. 2020;288:335–44. https://doi.org/10.1111/joim.13089.
118. Torjesen I. Covid-19: Middle aged women face greater risk of debilitating long term symptoms. BMJ. 2021;372:n829. https://doi.org/10.1136/bmj.n829.
119. Natri H, Garcia AR, Buetow KH, Trumble BC, Wilson MA. The pregnancy pickle: evolved immune compensation due to pregnancy underlies sex differences in human diseases. Trends Genet. 2019;35(7):478–88. https://doi.org/10.1016/j.tig.2019.04.008.
120. Khamsi R. Rogue antibodies could be driving severe COVID-19. Nature. 2021;590(7844):29–31. https://doi.org/10.1038/d41586-021-00149-1.
121. Steardo L, Steardo L Jr, Zorec R, Verkhratsky A. Neuroinfection may contribute to pathophysiology and clinical manifestations of COVID-19. Acta Physiol (Oxf). 2020;229(3):e13473. https://doi.org/10.1111/apha.13473.
122. Markus HS, Brainin M. COVID-19 and stroke—a global World Stroke Organization perspective. Int J Stroke. 2020;15(4):361–4. https://doi.org/10.1177/1747493020923472.
123. Minnelli N, Gibbs L, Larrivee J, Sahu KK. Challenges of maintaining optimal nutrition status in COVID-19 patients in intensive care settings. JPEN J Parenter Enteral Nutr. 2020;44(8):1439–46.
124. Dhatt SS, Kumar V, Neradi D, et al. Need for testing and supplementation of vitamin D3 after release of COVID-19 lockdown in patients with increased musculoskeletal pain. Indian J Orthop. 2021, 2021:1–4. https://doi.org/10.1007/s43465-021-00376-8.
125. Wang X, Sahu KK, Cerny J. Coagulopathy, endothelial dysfunction, thrombotic microangiopathy and complement activation: potential role of complement system inhibition in COVID-19. J Thromb Thrombolysis. 2021;51(3):657–62.
126. Dani M, Dirksen A, Taraborrelli P, Torocastro M, Panagopoulos D, Sutton R, Lim PB (2021) Autonomic dysfunction in 'long COVID': rationale, physiology and management strategies. Clin Med (Lond) 21(1):e63-e67.
127. Sterner RM, Sakemura R, Cox MJ, et al. GM-CSF inhibition reduces cytokine release syndrome and neuroinflammation but enhances CAR-T cell function in xenografts. Blood. 2019;133(7):697–709. https://doi.org/10.1182/blood-2018-10-881722.
128. Helms J, Kremer S, Merdji H, et al. Neurologic features in severe SARS-CoV-2 infection. N Engl J Med. 2020;382:2268–70.
129. Kandemirli SG, Dogan L, Sarikaya ZT, et al. Brain MRI findings in patients in the intensive care unit with COVID-19 Infection. Radiology. 2020;297(1):E232–5.
130. Nilsson A, Edner N, Albert J, Ternhag A. Fatal encephalitis associated with coronavirus OC43 in an immunocompromised child. Infect Dis (Auckl). 2020;52:419–22.
131. Ding Y, Wang H, Shen H, et al. The clinical pathology of severe acute respiratory syndrome (SARS): a report from China. J Pathol. 2003;200:282–9.
132. Lam DK, Dang D, Flynn AN, Hardt M, Schmidt BL. TMPRSS2, a novel membrane-anchored mediator in cancer pain. Pain. 2015;156(5):923–30.

2 Acute Manifestations of Neuro-COVID

2.1 Introduction. Overview on Clinical Manifestations of the Disease

The large number of symptoms of COVID-19 lead to multiple clinical pictures that require a precise taxonomy [1, 2]. In this uncertainty, the abundant medical literature produced can provide valuable help. In a study conducted on 20133 patients admitted to the hospital, the most common symptoms were cough (68.9%), fever (71.6%), and shortness of breath (71.2%) [3]. The authors found four clusters of symptoms; the most frequent ones concerned respiratory symptoms such as cough, sputum, shortness of breath, and fever; other clusters were musculoskeletal symptoms (myalgia, joint pain, headache, and fatigue), enteric symptoms (abdominal pain, vomiting, and diarrhea); less commonly, a mucocutaneous set of symptoms were grouped. An observational multi-center European study that enrolled patients (n = 1420) with a mild-to-moderate COVID-19 showed that the most common symptoms were headache (70.3%), loss of smell (70.2%), nasal obstruction (67.8%), cough (63.2%), asthenia (63.3%), myalgia (62.5%), rhinorrhea (60.1%), gustatory dysfunction (54.2%), sore throat (52.9%), and fever (45.4%) [4]. Furthermore, a systematic review and meta-analysis of the literature including a total of 2874 patients, showed different results with a higher incidence of fever (88.7%)—mainly in adults compared to children (92.8% vs 43.9%)—followed by cough (57.6%), and dyspnea (45.6%) [5]. Another systematic analysis found similar results with fever as the most prevalent clinical symptom (91.3%), followed by cough (67.7%), fatigue (51.0%), and dyspnea (30.4%) [6].

Notably, certain less common symptoms can represent the first manifestation of the disease. They can develop before the classic fever and respiratory symptoms, or be the unique clinical expression of COVID-19. These symptoms are deep vein thrombosis [7], diarrhea [8, 9], acute pancreatitis [10], acute hepatitis [11], and cutaneous manifestations, such as rash, urticaria, macular erythema, and others [12].

M. Cascella, E. De Blasio, *Features and Management of Acute and Chronic Neuro-Covid*, https://doi.org/10.1007/978-3-030-86705-8_2

A Cochrane review of the literature aimed at assessing the diagnostic accuracy of signs and symptoms of COVID-19 identified 16 studies including 7706 patients. Interestingly, 27 signs and symptoms were divided into four different categories: systemic, respiratory, gastrointestinal, and cardiovascular. The overall sensitivity was very low and the specificity was high. Since 6 symptoms (i.e., cough, sore throat, fever, myalgia/arthralgia, fatigue, and headache) were found with high sensitivity in at least one study, they should be considered red flags for suspect COVID-19 [13].

The matter becomes even more complicated when further variables come into play. About 25–30% of patients present comorbidities and this percentage increases to 60–90% among hospitalized patients, especially in intensive care unit (ICU) patients [14, 15]. The most common comorbidities include hypertension, diabetes, cardiovascular diseases, chronic obstructive pulmonary diseases, chronic kidney diseases, malignancy, and chronic liver disease, [3, 5, 6, 14]. Obesity has been also identified as a risk factor for the severity of the disease and poor outcome [15]. Age and sex seem to have a role in the prevalence of the symptoms, with the young patients more frequently showing ear, nose, and throat complaints and the elderly ones fatigue and fever. Concerning gender differences, loss of smell, headache, fatigue, and nasal obstruction were prevalent in females [4].

About the evolution and outcome of infected patients, a European study showed that of 1420 patients who completed the full evaluation, 116 needed hospitalization (8.1%) and the mean duration of COVID-19 symptoms (mild-to-moderate disease) was 11.5 ± 5.7 days [4]. A literature review showed that 17–35% of patients were treated in the ICU for acute respiratory failure and/or multiorgan failure [14]. In a prospective observational study conducted in 208 acute care hospitals, among 20133 inpatients with COVID-19, 17% required admission to high dependency or ICU, 55% received high flow oxygen at some point during their admission, 16% were treated with non-invasive ventilation, and 10% received invasive ventilation [3]. Other studies from the United States (US), Italy, and China showed a wide proportion range of critically ill among the inpatients (from 7% to 26%) [16–18]. The median time to in-hospital deterioration was 3 days and the length of stay increased with age [16].

The case-fatality rate varies among the countries, from 0.2 to 28.9% [19]. These differences could be explained by demographic reasons, as the proportion of older patients, the characteristics of healthcare systems, the differences in the number of people tested, the definition of COVID-19 related deaths, and testing strategies used to diagnose the disease [20]. Overall, the mortality rate of hospitalized patients ranges from 15% to 20%, up to 40% for those requiring ICU admission [14]. As expected, the mortality is higher for older patients and those with comorbidity [3].

Based on these premises, it is clear that COVID-19 is not just a respiratory disease. In other words, through direct and/or indirect viral damage (e.g., because of the inflammatory response), or during the evolution of the disease, all organs and systems can be potentially affected. In this context, the possibility that human coronaviruses (HCoVs) can produce neurological or psychiatric symptoms has been highlighted by studies conducted on the Severe Acute Respiratory Syndrome (SARS) and the Middle East Respiratory Syndrome (MERS). Both outbreaks were caused by viruses belonging to the family *Coronaviridae*, SARS-CoV and MERS-CoV, respectively. Cases of generalized seizures with the finding of cerebral spinal fluid (CSF) positivity for SARS-CoV were described [21]. Among the psychiatric consequences, depression, anxiety disorder, suicidal ideas, hallucinations, and behavioral disturbances were reported [22]. Besides, other HCoVs appear to be capable of producing neurological damage. For example, Nilsson et al. [23] reported a case of fatal encephalomyelitis associated with the HCoV OC43 in an immunocompromised child, despite absent respiratory involvement.

Concerning COVID-19, since the beginning of the pandemic, the first clinical reports indicated the presence of neurological symptoms and signs as part of the clinical manifestations of the disease. In a retrospective study in Wuhan (China), 36.4% of patients had neurologic symptoms, mainly in more severe patients. The neurological manifestations were divided into three categories: central, peripheral, and skeletal muscular symptoms. Central nervous system (CNS) manifestations such as dizziness, headache, impaired consciousness, acute cerebrovascular disease, ataxia, and seizure were more frequent (24.8% of cases), followed by peripheral problems (taste impairment, smell impairment, vision impairment, and nerve pain), and muscular symptoms (8.9% and 10.7%, respectively). The most common CNS symptoms were dizziness (16.8%) and headache (13.1%). Furthermore, the onset of symptoms was early for some peripheral (taste and smell impairment), skeletal muscle manifestations (myalgia and asthenia), and some CNS symptoms like dizziness and headache. On the contrary, impaired consciousness and acute cerebrovascular diseases appeared late in the course of the disease [24]. In another study, it was described that anosmia and ageusia were the unique presenting symptoms, in 3% of patients [14], and in a large international multicohort study on 3744 patients from 28 centers (13 countries), neurological manifestations were reported in 82% of hospitalized patients. The most common symptoms were headache, anosmia/ageusia; encephalopathy, coma, and stroke were also reported. Moreover, the presence of neurological signs and syndromes was associated with an increased risk of in-hospital death [25].

On these premises, in the context of COVID-19-related extrapulmonary clinical expressions, acute neurological and psychological/psychiatric manifestations configure a chapter of paramount importance. The term "neuro-COVID" is an umbrella term encompassing both acute manifestations and lasting symptoms or syndromes. In particular, the involvement of the CNS and/or PNS, as well as psychological/psychiatric problems can concern the acute phase of the disease, but also extend beyond its resolution. In the latter case, the phenomenology of neuro-COVID falls within post-acute clinical manifestations that are collectively referred to as "long-COVID" or "post-COVID."

Given that the pandemic is still ongoing and the ever-increasing amount of information on the subject, this chapter is aimed at presenting an overview of the acute manifestations of neuro-COVID. It is a particularly complex phenomenon. Pathophysiological, clinical, and epidemiological studies will help to clarify many doubts and questions that clinicians and scholars have on this issue. It is reasonable to think that it may take years to draw a complete picture of the problem.

2.2 Pathogenic Mechanisms

Growing evidence suggests a direct and indirect involvement of the CNS and peripheral nervous system (PNS) in the SARS-CoV-2 infection. Concerning the pathogenic mechanisms, it was shown that the angiotensin-converting enzyme 2 (ACE2), which is responsible for the interaction of the coronavirus with host cells, is expressed also in neurons, astrocytes, and oligodendrocytes of various areas of the brain like substantia nigra, ventricles, middle temporal gyrus, posterior cingulate cortex, and olfactory bulb [26, 27]. The virus could directly reach the CNS in retrograde entry through the olfactory epithelium or the retrograde transfer from nerve terminals (olfactory pathway) and cross, in turn, the damaged blood–brain barrier (BBB) [26, 28]. The trigeminal nerve, the glossopharyngeal nerve, and the vagus could be also involved in the nervous spreading. Additionally, SARS-CoV-2 could directly reach the nervous tissue by exploiting the hematogenous pathway, or cross the BBB carried by lymphatic cellular elements. The latter mechanism is called the "Trojan horse" pathway [29].

On the other hand, potential mechanisms of CNS and PNS involvement could be related to hypoxic injury, cerebrovascular injury, or be the effect of the immune-mediated injury. Hypoxic brain damage is the result of severe hypoxia because of acute respiratory failure, while the cytokine storm in the acute phase could be responsible for the immune-mediated injury and a dysregulated immune response. This exuberant immune-mediated inflammation could be responsible for central and peripheral autoimmune manifestations [27, 28]. Furthermore, neurologic involvement could result from sepsis and multiorgan failure, in the most severe cases [30].

Histological findings can help to clarify the mechanisms of the lesions and the occurrence of symptoms. A postmortem case series on 43 patients showed relatively mild alterations with areas of fresh ischemic lesions, in 14%, and astrogliosis, in 86% of patients. Activation of microglia and infiltration by cytotoxic T lymphocytes mainly in the brainstem and cerebellum was also demonstrated. Moreover, SARS-CoV-2 was detected in 53% of brains, cranial nerves, and brainstem, while there was no evidence of cerebral bleeding or small-vessel thrombosis and necrotizing lesions [31]. Another study showed a diffuse hypoxic injury in the cerebrum and cerebellum with loss of neurons in the cerebral cortex, hippocampus, and cerebellar Purkinje cell layer; no thrombi or vasculitis were found, while rare foci of perivascular lymphocytes and a focal leptomeningeal inflammation were detected; again, no abnormalities in the olfactory bulb were observed; the virus was detected in the brains of 5 patients [32]. Neuropathological findings from a case of acute disseminated encephalomyelitis showed mild brain swelling and hemorrhagic lesions; these lesions were disseminated throughout the cerebral hemispheric white matter and combined with intraparenchymal blood infiltration, and macrophages, peripherally [33].

Besides the potential SARS-CoV-2 neuroinvasion and neurotropism, as well as indirect damages produced by an excessive inflammatory and immune-mediated response of the hosts, other factors can probably contribute to the determinism of neurological complications in COVID-19. Some treatments and the environmental conditions adopted for COVID-19 patients, such as strict quarantine or the stay in ICU, could play a role in the development of neurological and psychiatric symptoms.

Despite these findings, the pathogenic underlying mechanism(s) of the neurological manifestations of COVID-19 need to be clarified. Further research is warranted for explaining if these phenomena can be considered as expressions of the viral damage or the result of complications involving the CNS and/or the PNS in light of the natural evolution of the disease. Overlapping mechanisms between direct/indirect viral attack and disease-related processes can probably occur (For more details on pathogenic mechanisms see Chap. 1).

2.3 Classification Approaches

There are many classifications of neurological involvement of COVID-19. These approaches concern:

- Pathogenetic mechanisms: direct damage, indirect injury (e.g., neuroinflammation and cytokine-related injury), disease-related (e.g., ischemic, multiorgan impairment)
- Location of symptoms: CNS, PNS, and skeletal muscular manifestations
- Onset time of the clinical presentations (infective and post-infective complications)

Yu et al. [34] suggested a classification based on the pathophysiology of the symptoms, identifying four categories:

1. CNS direct invasion including viral meningitis/encephalitis
2. PNS direct invasion featuring hyposmia and/or hypogeusia
3. Systemic response leading to hypoxic injury, coagulopathy, and inflammatory response like encephalopathy, and cerebrovascular diseases.
4. Post-infection immune dysfunction. This group encompasses acute disseminated encephalomyelitis (ADEM); acute necrotizing encephalitis (ANE); acute necrotizing myelitis (ANM); Guillain-Barré syndrome (GBS) and its variants.

Furthermore, Nersesjan et al. [35] proposed to assign the neurological complications to one of the following mechanisms:

1. Direct viral invasion:
   (a) Evidence of SARS-CoV-2 detected in CSF or evidence of SARS-CoV-2-specific intrathecal antibody production.
   (b) No other explanatory pathogen or cause was found.

2. Immune-mediated mechanisms:
   (a) Neurological disease onset within 6 weeks of acute infection.
   (b) No evidence of other commonly associated causes including recent or concomitant viral infections.
   (c) Evidence of immune-mediated mechanisms, such as inflammatory lesions on magnetic resonance imaging (MRI) and/or CSF pleocytosis or oligoclonal bands and/or brain pathology findings.
3. Complications secondary to critical illness, management-related, or other causes:
   (a) Other more likely causes, such as delirium, hypoxia, sepsis, metabolic derangement, or other complications to critical illness (e.g., septic or hypoxic encephalopathy).
   (b) No signs of disease mechanism 1 or 2 after investigation with brain imaging, electroencephalography (EEG), or CSF study.
4. Insufficiently investigated:
   (a) No explainable cause found.
   (b) CSF study and/or neuroimaging not able to confirm or dismiss 1 or 2 disease mechanisms.

A simple and effective approach refers to clinical presentations. The German Society of Neurology published recommendations and statements about the following clinical manifestations: encephalopathy, meningoencephalitis, GBS, acute inflammatory demyelinating polyneuritis (AIDP), ADEM, stroke, epilepsy, chemosensory disturbance, neuromuscular diseases, and PNS diseases [36].

The clinical distinction based on the location of the underlying lesion appears to be a simple and accepted classification criterion. In a retrospective observational study from 46 hospitals in France on COVID-19 patients ($n = 222$) with neurological manifestations, the authors classified the neurological manifestations in CNS and PNS clinical expressions [37]. They also defined each clinical picture:

- Stroke: patients with sudden neurologic deficit related to an acute vascular lesion on MRI or computed tomography (CT) scan, or n patients with a transient focal deficit and normal MRI (transient ischemic attack) or in those with cerebral venous thrombosis.
- Encephalitis: an altered mental status lasting 24 h along with one of the following criteria: white blood cell count (WBC) in CSF less than 5/mm^3; or presence of a compatible acute lesion on brain MRI.
- Encephalopathy: an altered mental status lasting more than 24 h that could be associated with seizure and/or focal neurologic signs in the absence of criteria for encephalitis and if encephalopathy could not be accounted for by another cause, such as toxic or metabolic factors, according to the reporting clinician.
- GBS: according to standard diagnostic criteria, progressive motor weakness of more than one limb, areflexia, symptoms progression, relative symmetry, mild sensory symptoms or signs, cranial nerve involvement, autonomic dysfunction, absence of fever at the onset, CSF protein elevated and cells count of 10 or fewer mononuclear leukocytes/mm^3.

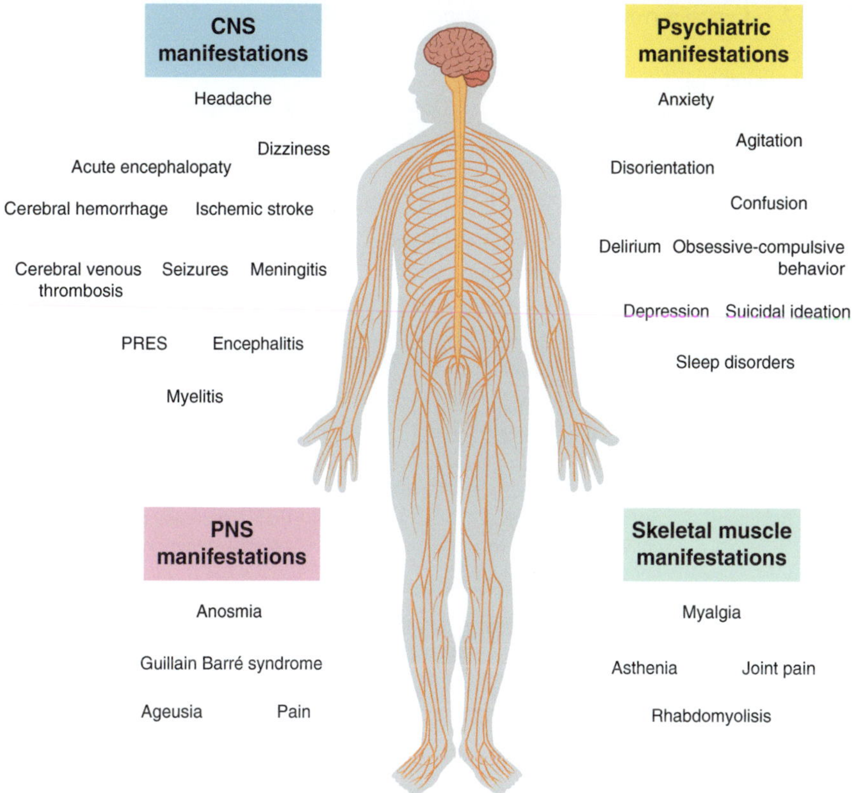

Fig. 2.1 Acute manifestations of neuro-COVID

- Acute meningitis: meningeal syndrome (head stiffness, headache, fever) without encephalitic course and CSF WBC counts less than 5/mm^3.
- Other: neurologic manifestations that did not meet any of these criteria.

Following this approach, in this chapter, a simple descriptive model based on the location of clinical manifestations, is adopted. Neurological manifestations are divided into CNS, and PNF issues. Moreover, skeletal muscular manifestations and several acute psychological/psychiatric problems are also encompassed in the acute neuro-COVID (Fig. 2.1).

2.4 Central Nervous System Manifestations

This group encompasses clinical manifestations of varying severity, incidence, and weight. These complications are reported in Table 2.1.

Table 2.1 Central nervous system manifestations of COVID-19

Clinical manifestation [Ref.]	Features	Occurrence	Pathogenesis
Headache [25, 38–43]	Tension-type or migraine without aura, migraine-like headache (less commonly); long-lasting duration and analgesic resistance	4–23%	Neuroinflammation, activation of the trigeminovascular system, stressful conditions
Dizziness [24, 28, 41, 43]	Combined with headache (and tinnitus), it is often observed in earlier disease	8–17%	Vascular damage?
Acute encephalopathy [13, 19, 24–26, 38, 40, 41, 43–50]	Delirium or decreased level of consciousness up to coma with or without seizures and extrapyramidal signs	3.8–69%	Alteration of neurotransmitters; toxic metabolites; proinflammatory cytokines
Posterior reversible encephalopathy syndrome (PRES) [51–57]	Altered consciousness, seizures, headaches and visual disturbances	1.1–3.9%	The binding of the virus to ACE2 receptors causes a fluctuation of blood pressure and weakening of endothelial layer, leading to a dysfunction of cerebral autoregulation and altered BBB function with hypoperfusion of the posterior circulation
Seizures [36, 58–64]	Focal motor, tonic-clonic, convulsive status epilepticus, and non-convulsive status epilepticus	0.6–2.8%	Alteration of neurotransmitters; toxic metabolites; proinflammatory cytokines; coagulation alterations; electrolytes disturbances
Acute cerebrovascular diseases [25, 65, 66]	Ischemic strokes, cerebral hemorrhages, CVT	1.4–6% (ischemic strokes 87%; hemorrhages 11.6%; CVT 0.5%)	Hypercoagulability, high systemic inflammatory response, vascular endothelial injury, alteration of cerebral autoregulation and hemodynamic lability, cardiac injury resulting in cerebral embolism

Table 2.1 (continued)

Clinical manifestation [Ref.]	Features	Occurrence	Pathogenesis
Meningitis and encephalitis [25, 36, 67–74]	Agitation, disorientation, meningeal rigidity, photophobia, hallucinations, reduced level of consciousness, and focal status epilepticus	0.5%	Intracranial cytokine storm or Para-infectious demyelination
Acute myelitis [25, 50, 75–79]	Mostly transverse myelitis, with different degrees of paresis, up to quadri/paraplegia, accompanied by sensitive and sphincter dysfunction	Case reports; case series; 18 patients in a review	Damage linked to cytokines released by inflammatory storms or immune-mediated mechanisms

Abbreviations: *ACE2* angiotensin-converting enzyme2, *CVT* cerebral venous thrombosis, *BBB* blood-brain barrier

2.4.1 Headache and Dizziness

Headache, a non-specific symptom of many diseases, is one of the most common symptoms of COVID-19. It is often associated with fever [26], but can also be a presenting symptom of the disease. In a retrospective study, the headache was the most commonly reported symptom with the appearance during the first 3 days in 62.3% of patients and a median duration of 4 days [38]. A scoping review and meta-analysis of 61 studies and 59,254 patients showed that headache was the fifth most common symptom (12%, 95% CI: 4%–23%) after fever (82%), cough (61%), muscle aches/fatigue (36%), and dyspnea (26%) [39]. In another analysis, the prevalence of headache was 10%, and no statistical difference was found between severe and non-severe patients ($p = 0.78$), survived and non-survived ($p = 0.23$), and ICU patients versus non-ICU patients ($p = 0.87$) [40]. Moreover, in a systematic review and meta-analysis on neurologic characteristics in COVID-19 ($n = 7559$), the overall pooled prevalence of the symptom was 10.9% (95% CI: 8.62–13.51) [41]. In a study on the general population, a periodic longitudinal questionnaire was administered to 21,359 subjects regardless of a history of COVID-19 infection or test. Headache was reported in 71.4% of hospitalized and 79.1% of non-hospitalized patients during the acute phase of the disease [80]. In the international multicohort study on 3055 hospitalized patients, the headache was the most common self-reported symptom (37%) [25].

Clinically, the headache does not present typical characteristics. The severity usually varies from moderate (dull headache) to severe and could be related to the severity of infection. It has been reported as tension-type or migraine without aura, less frequently as migraine-like headache with throbbing or pulsing sensations and aggravation with head/neck movements [40]. Notably, disabling headache can persist (weeks/months) after COVID-19 resolution. In this case, headache is encompassed among the clinical manifestation of long-COVID.

In a web-based survey on COVID-19 positive and negative subjects, the headache was more closely associated with anosmia/ageusia and gastrointestinal complaints. Bilateral headache, long-lasting duration, and analgesic resistance were more frequent in COVID-19 positive patients. Most patients with a previous headache reported that the new headache was partially or totally different from the usual one and mainly with pulsating characteristics. Furthermore, the respondents reported that the most frequent headache triggers were infection itself and stress, followed by received drugs, wearing masks, and social isolation [42].

The symptom can also be used for disease diagnosis (sentinel symptoms). In a bundle proposed for determining if a patient presenting in primary care or hospital outpatient settings has COVID-19 disease, the headache was one of the six trigger flags. The analysis showed a low sensitivity (0.03–0.71 for hospital outpatient clinics and 0.15 for hospital inpatients) and a good specificity (0.78–0.98 for hospital outpatient clinics and 0.97 for hospital inpatients) [13].

About pathogenesis, the proposed mechanism underlying headache is neuroinflammatory, suggesting a release of cytokines and chemokines during the development of the disease [26]. The effect is the activation of the trigeminovascular system. Furthermore, the concomitant anosmia can suggest a direct involvement of SARS-CoV-2.

Since during COVID-19 headache could be caused by more serious conditions, it is mandatory a closely monitoring of patient's consciousness and a careful evaluation of any potential cause for excluding the onset of more serious complications such as meningitis, encephalitis, and intracranial hypertension [26, 39].

Dizziness is a minor symptom associated with COVID-19. It is present in different reports and its pathogenesis is not well understood [27]. In a retrospective study, it was present in 16.8% of patients with a nonstatistical difference between severe and non-severe infection (19.3 vs. 15.1%, $p = 0.42$) [24]. A multi-center study through an online questionnaire investigated the presence of tinnitus and equilibrium disorders (vertigo/dizziness); of 185 COVID-19 patients, 18.4% reported balance disorders, of whom 94.1% dizziness and 5.9% acute vertigo attacks, while 23.2% reported tinnitus after disease diagnosis [43]. In another study on the general population, Cirulli et al. [80] found dizziness in in 38% of COVID-19 patients, and 10.9% of non-COVID-19 ones. Other studies showed a lower prevalence (8.77%) of dizziness, although its occurrence in the earlier disease was better underlined [41]. Since the inner ear structures are susceptible to ischemia due to their characteristics of terminal vasculature, vascular damage underlying the disorder was suggested [43]. Vestibular neuritis can be also assumed.

Practical Therapeutic Suggestions
- Symptomatic therapy (e.g., paracetamol or ibuprofen).
- Evaluate potentially associated symptoms and signs (e.g., focal neurologic
- symptoms).
- Vestibular rehabilitation can be suggested for dizziness, especially if persistent and associated with other disorders (e.g., nausea).

2.4.2 Acute Encephalopathy

Disorders of consciousness are described by many reports. They vary from an altered consciousness content (confusion and/or delirium) to reduction of consciousness level (somnolence, stupor, coma) [24, 80]. These disorders are also referred to as an acute confusional state, acute brain dysfunction, or failure. Therefore, it would be appropriate to refer to the recommendations recently provided by a consensus of 10 scientific societies. According to this consensus statement, the term "acute encephalopathy" indicates a rapid developing (less than 4 weeks but usually within hours to few days) pathobiological brain process which is clinically expressed as either subsyndromal delirium or delirium or decreased level of consciousness up to coma and may have additional features, such as seizures and extrapyramidal signs [45].

In the Chou's et al. [25] study, among the 3744 hospitalized patients, acute encephalopathy was the most common clinical sign with an incidence of 49%; on the other hand, coma was described in 17% of those. Both encephalopathy and coma were associated with an increase of in-hospital mortality.

Some predisposing factors could be already present at the time of infection. They encompass advanced age, preexisting cognitive impairment, and malnutrition. Other factors such as infections, electrolyte alterations (especially hypo/hypernatremia), renal and hepatic insufficiency, and hypo/hyperglycemia can occur during the evolution of the disease [26].

Three main pathophysiological mechanisms could underlie the impaired consciousness. These processes are not dissimilar to those underlying delirium and other manifestations of acute brain dysfunction in ICU [47–49]:

- Alteration of neurotransmitters caused by the use of anticholinergic or dopaminergic medications.
- Accumulation of toxic metabolites associated with organ failure.
- Systemic inflammatory storm due to the release of proinflammatory cytokines.

In COVID-19, other conditions, including severe hypoxia and cerebral hypoperfusion, could explain an altered level of consciousness seen in these patients [27, 28, 36]. In some cases, altered mental status could be related to rare complications of a viral infection such as ANE [41]. Since pathophysiology can be difficult to explain, the correlation with the clinic can offer important information. In a case series on 55 patients, encephalopathy was classified based on its severity:

- No encephalopathy: fully awake, preserved sustained and basic attention, without neuropsychiatric disturbances or psychomotor slowing.
- Mild encephalopathy: awake or easily arousable patient, with preserved basic attention but impaired sustained attention. Patients with preserved sustained attention and level of consciousness, but presenting psychiatric, behavioral symptoms, or psychomotor slowing were also included in this group.
- Moderate encephalopathy: awake or easily arousable patient, with impaired basic and sustained attention.
- Severe encephalopathy: comatose patients or patients requiring vigorous stimuli to be aroused. Patients with severe psychomotor agitation were also included in this group.

In this series, 21.8% had no encephalopathy, 21.8% mild, 32.6% moderate, and 23.6% severe encephalopathy. Among all the cases, changes of behavior were present in 9% (especially in mild encephalopathy); psychomotor agitation in 2%; disorientation in 14% (mainly in mild cases). Other features such as quadriparesis, myoclonus, and the appearance of seizures, were found in 2–12% of cases. Neuroimaging showed mostly non-specific changes and in 1 case a demyelination picture. While the CSF examination showed elevated WBC in 9%, it was negative for oligoclonal bands. Again, interleukin (IL)-6 was quantified in 7 patients and was found elevated in three severe patients. The authors concluded that in COVID-19 patients, although the direct viral invasion was not proved, and the immune-mediated CNS response and systemic cytokine storm could be responsible for the occurrence of the manifestations, other factors, such as the use of sedatives and multiorgan failure, could play an important role. In turn, the precise underlying mechanisms remain to be clarified [81].

In a retrospective case series the "acute encephalopathy," referred to as impaired consciousness, was present in 7.5% of patients and occurred late in the course of the hospital stay; it was more common in patients with severe infection compared with nonsevere infections (14.8% vs. 2.4%, $p < 0.001$) [24]. In another report on ICU patients with COVID-19-associated acute respiratory distress syndrome (ARDS), agitation was detected in 69% using confusion assessment method (CAM)-ICU scale, and dysexecutive syndrome—dysregulation of executive functions due to frontal lobe damage featuring emotional, motivational, and behavioral symptoms as well as cognitive deficits—occurred in 36% of patients. Agitation was mainly shown after the discontinuation of sedation and neuromuscular blockade [44]. In a systematic review and meta-analysis on neurologic characteristics in COVID-19, the overall pooled prevalence of consciousness disturbance was 3.8% (95% CI: 0.16–12.04) [41]. Finally, in a recent review of 42 records, encephalopathy was common in both older and more severe patients with advanced disease. Common clinical features were confusion, agitation, delirium, and coma although in some cases the patients showed additional clinical manifestations such as seizures, headache, or extrapyramidal signs. The most common MRI findings were cortical or subcortical white matter T2/fluid-attenuated inversion recovery (FLAIR) signal hyperintensity; nevertheless, in some cases, MRI showed the features of ANE or ADEM. Most of the patients improved during the course of the disease [50].

In summary, due to the lack of a precise diagnostic criterion adopted in the various studies, it is difficult to establish the numerical entity of the problem.

Practical Therapeutic Suggestions

- The various pathologic mechanisms and the heterogeneity of symptomatology make it difficult to identify a specific treatment.
- It is suggested a general control of homeostasis, such as hydro-electrolytic equilibrium and body temperature, and the use of specific treatments, such as neuroleptics for psychic symptoms, and antiepileptics for the control of seizures.
- Antivirals, such as acyclovir and lopinavir/ritonavir, corticosteroid, IV immunoglobulins, have been also suggested.

2.4.3 Posterior Reversible Encephalopathy Syndrome

Posterior reversible encephalopathy syndrome (PRES) is characterized by a neurological symptomatology that includes altered consciousness, seizures, headaches, and visual disturbances. In some cases, focal deficits, such as hemiparesis and speaking difficulty, have been reported. Among patients undergoing imaging studies, the prevalence of PRES has been reported between 1.1% and 3.9%. This syndrome is caused by vasogenic edema linked to alteration of cerebrovascular autoregulation, and endothelial dysfunction leading to preferential hypoperfusion of the posterior circulation [51]. The radiological findings of brain comprise, on non-contrast brain CT, hypodense lesions in areas of the posterior cerebral circulation and, on MRI, areas of vasogenic edema as hypointense areas on the T1-weighted MRI and hyperintense areas on the T2-weighted/FLAIR MRI sequences, and lack of diffusion restriction [51].

The first reports of PRES described two patients with acute kidney failure and moderate fluctuating hypertension. An altered consciousness during the weaning from mechanical ventilation was reported in both subjects. MRI showed axial T2 FLAIR hyperintensity, involving the subcortical white matter of occipital lobes and/or posterior temporal lobes and cerebellar hemisphere, with effacement of the adjacent sulci. Further, axial susceptibility weighted imaging (SWI) showed convexal subarachnoid hemorrhage, in a case, and petechial hemorrhage, in the other one. Diffusion-weighted imaging (DWI) and T1 post-contrast imaging were unremarkable. The patients were treated with antihypertensives with a gradual recovery of symptomatology. Probably, the endothelial dysfunction in COVID-19 patients could induce PRES at a lower level of blood pressure. It suggests a stricter control of blood pressure [52].

Other four cases of PRES were reported in four patients with acute kidney injury and elevated blood pressure. All the patients were encephalopathic, showing confusion, and agitation, and in two cases there was epileptiform activity. The CT findings were characterized by bilateral hypoattenuation involving the bilateral occipital or parieto-occipital white matter. Again, the MRI showed confluent T2 hyperintensities, without diffusion restriction or susceptibility hypointensity in the same regions in all patients but one. All the patients improved with blood pressure and seizure control. The authors postulated that tumor necrosis factor (TNF)-α, associated with cytokine storm, could increase vascular permeability and upregulate vascular endothelial growth factor in the setting of hypoxia, leading to vasogenic edema. Furthermore, the authors underlined that also some drugs used for the treatment of COVID-19, such as hydroxychloroquine, could play a role in the pathogenesis of PRES [53].

In a case series from Italy of four patients with agitation and spatial disorientation and one case of generalized seizure after weaning from mechanical ventilation, the MRI study showed multiple areas (from punctiform to some millimeters in extension) hyperintense on T2-weighted, and FLAIR images, located in the parietal, occipital, and frontal regions. On diffusion MRI, all but two lesions were characterized by the absence of apparent diffusion coefficient changes. A subtle contrast enhancement was detected in a cortical lesion. Based on the prevalent cortical involvement and diffusion MRI pattern, not typical of this syndrome, a multifactorial mechanism related to a dysregulation of vasomotor reactivity, with transient vasoconstriction, endothelial dysfunction, and impaired microcirculation, can be hypothesized [54]. Other six cases with characteristic symptomatology were described. In particular, five patients needed ICU admission and developed seizures during the weaning from mechanical ventilation. It can be suggested that the restoration of normal cerebral oxygenation can induce an irritative activity of the cerebral cortex during the passage to normal breathing [55].

The action of the massive cytokine release, leading to the breakdown of the BBB and coagulation impairment is a potential mechanism for explaining the pathogenesis of PRES. It can explain some atypical presentations of PRES that have been also described in the literature. They featured lethargy and confusion, and MRI imaging showing areas of vasogenic edema predominantly in parieto-occipital regions associated with diffuse petechiae or intraparenchymal hematoma [56, 57].

Practical Therapeutic Suggestions

The treatment consists of:

- Supportive care with hydration.
- Correction of electrolyte disturbances.
- Monitoring of airway and ventilation. Intubation in patients with altered mental status.

- Strict control of blood pressure. Since the rapid decrease in blood pressure could cause cerebral, coronary, and renal ischemia, the goal is to reduce blood pressure between 105 and 125 mmHg, without exceeding 25% of this reduction in the first hour. Calcium antagonists such as nimodipine, nicardipine, and verapamil are first-line treatments; they can also prevent cerebral vasospasm. Beta-blockers (e.g., labetalol) can be also used. Sodium nitroprusside, hydralazine, and diazoxide are second-line drugs. Nitroglycerin should be avoided due to its vasodilator effect (increase of the cerebral edema). Fenoldopam mesylate, a selective dopamine 1 agonist that induces renal vasodilation, can be also used.
- Treatment of seizures. It is similar to that of other epileptic seizures. Intravenous benzodiazepines (e.g., lorazepam or diazepam) are used as first-line therapy. As second-line, phenytoin or valproate, especially in status epilepticus, or phenobarbital. Propofol, pentobarbital, and midazolam are used in refractory seizures. Magnesium sulfate is used in pregnant women.
- Control of the trigger (e.g., withdrawal of cancer chemotherapy or immunosuppressive agents)

2.4.4 Seizures

Among clinical manifestations of COVID-19, new onset of a focal or generalized seizure and status epilepticus were reported in the literature. In an extensive database on 40,469 COVID-19 patients (9086 had neuropsychiatric manifestation), seizures were reported in 258 patients (0.6% of all patients and 2.8% of patients with neurologic manifestations) [58]. In a recent retrospective study on 439 cases of COVID-19, 4.3% of patients showed new-onset seizures without underlying pathology, while 2 (0.46%) had previously controlled epilepsy with breakthrough seizures. Furthermore, in 14 patients (3.18%) there was a primary pathology such as stroke, encephalitis, or brain tumor explaining the occurrence of seizures [59].

The etiology of COVID-19-related seizures is multifactorial. It was suggested that comorbidities like diabetes, and renal failure, clinical features including hypoxia, cardiovascular failure, and multiorgan failure, specific neurological complications such as stroke, and encephalitis, as well as some medications used during COVID-19 disease, could trigger an episode of seizure [60]. In particular, the central role of the activated microglia has been emphasized. After the invasion of CNS, the virus could trigger reactive astrogliosis with the release of proinflammatory cytokines ILβ1 and TNF-α leading to an increase of glutamate and a decrease of gamma-aminobutyric acid (GABA) in the cerebral cortex and hippocampus; the coexistent hypoxia could further increase the damage; systemic cytokines could enter the brain tissue through disrupted BBB and, therefore, this last mechanism could also promote the migration of proteins in the cerebral tissue with an alteration of osmotic balance [61]. Furthermore, inflammatory cytokines play another role through mitochondrial dysfunction with alteration of the normal electrical activity within neuronal functioning and synaptic transmission [61]. In COVID-19 patients, other two mechanisms are potentially involved in the onset of epilepsy. The former concerns coagulation abnormalities that can cause acute ischemia generating seizures by increasing extracellular glutamate concentrations, impaired ion channel function, and BBB damage; the latter mechanism regards electrolytes disturbances, mainly expressed as hyponatremia, hypocalcemia, and hypomagnesemia [61].

Seizures can present as focal motor, tonic-clonic, convulsive status epilepticus, and non-convulsive status epilepticus [60]. Since patients could develop a subclinical seizure and a status epilepticus, in the clinical evaluation of depressed consciousness this condition should not be overlooked [62].

In addition to new-onset seizures, special attention should be paid to the course of COVID-19 in patients diagnosed with epilepsy before infection. In this regard, a cross-sectional observational study estimated the incidence and case-fatality rate of COVID-19 in patients with active epilepsy. It was demonstrated that compared to the population without epilepsy, the cumulative incidence of COVID-19 in patients with epilepsy was higher (1.2% vs. 0.5%). Additionally, the total case- fatality rate was higher in patients with active epilepsy compared to patients without active epilepsy (23.8% vs. 3.6%; $p < 0.001$) and considering only hospitalized patients (50% vs. 16.1%; $p = 0.005$). The authors stated that these results could be explained by the higher vulnerability of patients with epilepsy [63]. Finally, in these patients, other potential mechanisms (e.g., the interactions between antiepileptic drugs and their effects on the immune system) could contribute to the worsening of the outcome and should be carefully considered in the treatment of epileptic patients with COVID-19 [64].

Practical suggestions for the management of COVID-19 patients with seizures were released by the German Society of Neurology [36]:

- If epileptic seizures, or a status epilepticus, occur in patients with COVID-19 disease, it should be clarified whether it is a first-time seizure or a recurrence of previously known epilepsy.
- In the case of unclear disturbance of consciousness, an EEG should be performed to detect and localize activity typical for epilepsy and to detect or exclude a non-convulsive status epilepticus.
- The treatment of seizures, or status epilepticus, should be performed according to the respective guidelines.
- Contraindications and interactions of anticonvulsants with substances used for COVID-19 disease should be taken into account.
- In patients with known fever-associated seizures, nonsteroidal anti-inflammatory drugs (NSAIDs) or paracetamol should be given.

Practical Therapeutic Suggestions

According to the German Society of Neurology [36]:

- If epileptic seizures, or a status epilepticus, occur in patients with COVID-19, it should be clarified whether it is a first-time seizure or a recurrence of previously known epilepsy.
- In the case of unclear disturbance of consciousness, an EEG should be performed to detect and localize activity typical for epilepsy and to detect or exclude a non-convulsive status epilepticus.
- The treatment of seizures, or status epilepticus, should be performed according to the respective guidelines.
- Contraindications and interactions of anticonvulsants with substances used for COVID-19 should be taken into account.
- In patients with known fever-associated seizures, nonsteroidal anti-inflammatory drugs (NSAIDs) or paracetamol should be given.

2.4.5 Acute Cerebrovascular Diseases

Acute cerebrovascular disease is one of the most serious neurologic complications seen in COVID-19 (Fig. 2.2). The incidence varies from 1% to 5% in hospitalized patients, and up to 6% in the setting of ICU patients [67, 82–84]. In a systematic review and meta-analysis from two studies with a total number of 435 total cases, the overall pooled prevalence of acute cerebrovascular disease was 4.4% (95% CI: 1.92–7.91) [41]. In another international multicohort study ($n = 3744$), acute stroke was reported in 6% of patients [25], and in a recent analysis ($n = 108{,}571$) in 1.4% [65].

Data provided by some recent literature reviews can help to characterize the number of these complications. It seems that cerebrovascular diseases affect more frequently [41, 84, 85]:

- COVID 19 older patients with severe coronavirus disease
- Individuals with one or more cardiovascular risk factors
- Those with previous cerebrovascular disease

A systematic review showed that in 47.2% of COVID-19 patients affected by ischemic disease during the infection, at least two vascular risk factors were found; moreover, in a third of patients one risk factor was present, and in about one-fifth there was no risk factor. The mean age was 64.16 ± 14.73 years (range 27–92 years). Among the risk factors, there were mostly coronary artery disease (10.2%), and previous cerebrovascular events (5.8%) [86]. Concerning the age, in a series of 23 patients, a binary regression logistic modeling showed that age was the only independent predictive factor of unfavorable outcome (OR = 1.5, 95% CI:

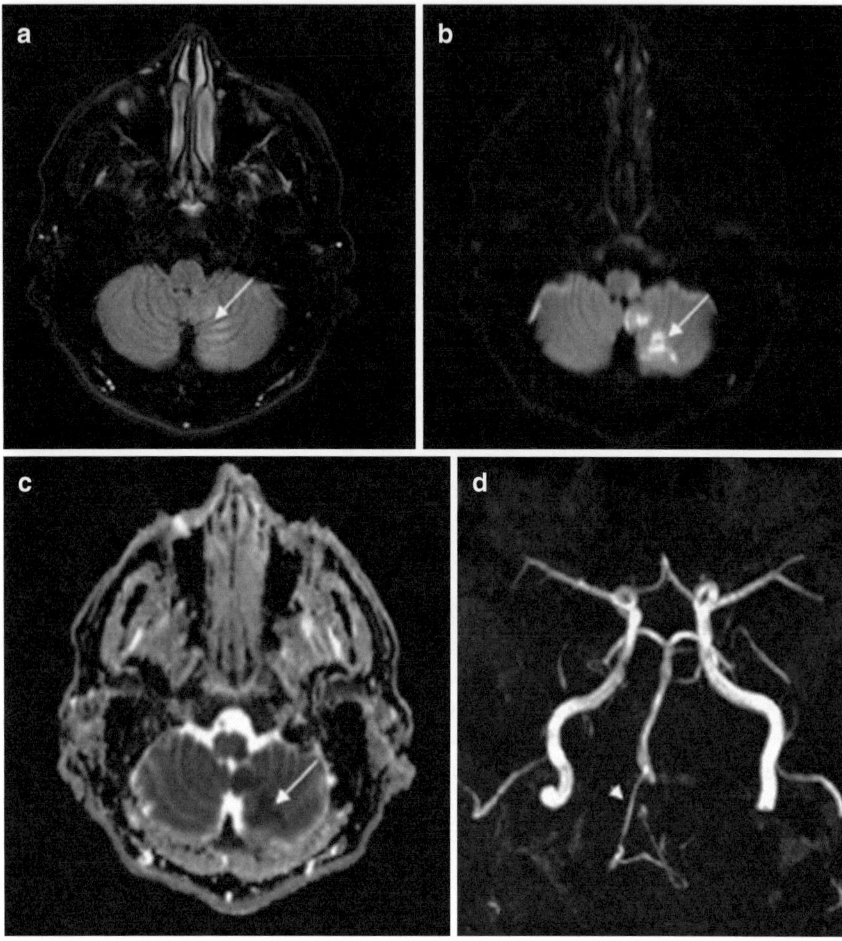

Fig. 2.2 COVID-19 patient with a stroke in the left vertebral artery (Wallenberg syndrome). The MRI shows in the fluid-attenuated inversion recovery (FLAIR) T2 sequence (**a**) a slight hyperintensity of the signal (white arrow), which in the diffusion-weighted imaging (DWI) sequence (**b**) appears hyperintense, and with reduced diffusion values in the apparent diffusion coefficient (ADC) maps (as in acute ischemia). In the MRI angiography scan (**c**, **d**), the right vertebral artery (arrowhead) is visible, but the left vertebral artery not

1.012–2.225; $p = 0.043$). Of note, the cut-off was 63 years (AUC 0.907; CI 0.78–1; $p = 0.003$) (sensitivity 82.4%, specificity 100%) [87]. In a single-center retrospective study on older COVID-19 inpatients ($n = 265$), the incidence of ischemic or hemorrhagic stroke was 4.15%. A higher prevalence of smoking (27.3% vs. 4.8%; $p = 0.019$), and history of previous stroke (45.5% vs. 13.8%; $p = 0.014$) was found. Again, no differences were observed for other comorbidities, frailty, and the severity of COVID-19 [88]. In their analysis of 108,571 patients, Nannoni et al. [65] confirmed these findings. Notably, COVID-19 patients at increased risk of cerebrovascular disease were older, more likely to have hypertension, diabetes mellitus, coronary artery disease, and a severe clinical picture. Furthermore, compared to stroke patients without infection, the population of stroke patients with COVID-19 was younger, with higher National Institutes of Health Stroke Scale (NIHSS), high frequency of large vessel occlusion, and higher in-hospital mortality [65].

In a retrospective observational study on 214 patients, Mao et al. [24] found acute cerebrovascular events in 2.8% of patients; compared to non-severe patients, the incidence was higher in the severely infected population (5.7% vs. 0.8%, $p = 0.03$); five of the six reported events (83.3%) were ischemic strokes, and one was hemorrhagic. In another study, 1.4% of patients developed cerebrovascular disease, of whom 73.9% ischemic and 21.7% were hemorrhagic [87]. These findings were confirmed in other investigations. Collantes et al. [89] showed that among all the neurological disorders and complications cerebrovascular problems were the most frequent (69.7%). Moreover, ischemic stroke was more frequent (78.2%), followed by hemorrhagic stroke (17.3%), and cerebral venous sinus thrombosis (4.3%). These findings were confirmed also in analysis on a large number of patients, showing that among the patients with cerebrovascular lesions ischemic stroke was the most common (87.4%), while intracerebral hemorrhage (11.6%), and cerebral venous thrombosis (0.5%) were less common [65].

Concerning clinical presentation, the majority of patients with an ischemic stroke presented with typical COVID-19 symptoms including fever (63.7%), acute respiratory symptoms (76.0%), and dyspnea (58.6%) [84]. Nevertheless, Fraiman et al. [86] reported that up to 15% of patients were asymptomatic. Although the mean duration from the first symptoms of infection and the onset of the neurological symptoms was 9–15 days [41, 84, 88], interestingly it was described that patients may present neurologic symptoms (e.g., hemiplegia) without any fever or upper respiratory tract symptom [24].

Similarly, the literature offers other contradictory data on this neurological complication. It was demonstrated, for example, that stroke and other neurovascular issues can also affect younger COVID-19 patients [83]. In a retrospective cohort study of 32 consecutive COVID-19 patients admitted with ischemic stroke, the median age was lower than contemporary stroke controls without COVID-19 ($p = 0.001$) [90]. Interestingly, younger patients seem to have some common features:

- No classical risk factors.
- Early onset of neurological symptoms.
- Occlusion of large vessels.

These features could suggest a central role of COVID-19 pathophysiology in determining the stroke [53]. In other words, neurovascular complications are produced directly by the disease, through direct and/or indirect viral damage, rather than being the consequence of exacerbated preexisting factors.

Complex pathogenesis, linked to systemic cytokine storm, direct immune-mediated mechanism, virus-induced vasculitis, and activation of systemic coagulopathy, could explain these findings [91]. Indeed, the etiology of cerebrovascular disorders during COVID-19 is multifactorial. An exaggerated inflammatory response with the release of large amounts of cytokines, such as IL1, IL6, and TNF-α, could cause the expression of tissue factor (TF) by endothelial and mononuclear cells, and thrombin generation, determining, finally, a procoagulant state [92]. Another potential mechanism could be linked to the endothelial dysfunction due to direct binding of SARS-CoV-2 to ACE2 receptors on the endothelial cell. This mechanism could explain some of the characteristics of stroke in the course of the disease [67, 83]. The detection of anticardiolipin IgA, and antiphospholipid IgA and IgM antibodies directed against β2 -glycoprotein-1 and lupus anticoagulant in some patients, suggests other possible prothrombotic mechanisms [93]. Furthermore, the inflammatory state could destabilize the atherosclerotic plaques increasing the risk of thromboembolism, as well as cardioembolism when in presence of cardiac arrhythmias or cardiac failure [92]. Finally, the downregulation of ACE2 expression could cause an imbalance of the renin–angiotensin system, with higher levels of Angiotensin II and increased vascular resistance, leading to a condition of elevated blood pressure and systemic inflammation with an increased risk of hemorrhagic stroke [92].

Some features of ischemic stroke are common in COVID-19 patients: large vessel occlusion, involvement of multiple territories, and the thrombosis of rarely affected arteries, such as the pericallosal artery [82]. Nevertheless, up to 40% of strokes were defined as cryptogenic, with a radiological appearance of embolic origin [82]. About the vascular territory involved and extension, it was reported a higher prevalence of the anterior vascular territory (81.7%), large vessel occlusion in 79.6%, and multiple infarctions in 42.5% of cases [65]. A case of massive bilateral stroke has been described in a patient admitted with the respiratory symptoms of COVID-19 who showed an initial drowsiness progressed to deep coma; brain CT angiogram illustrated occlusion in both the left internal carotid artery and the right middle cerebral artery [94].

Hemorrhagic stroke can be massive and, usually, it is featured by intracerebral hemorrhage (ICH) with complete involvement of a hemisphere, or it appears as multiple hematomas occurring in supra and infra-tentorial locations. Intracranial bleeding can also manifest as non-traumatic subarachnoid hemorrhage (SAH). In about one-fifth of hemorrhagic strokes, the simultaneous presence of ICH and SAH was observed [82]. It was shown that intraparenchymal lobar hematoma was the most frequent radiological finding, followed by bilateral location [65]. Hemorrhage could be also a transformation of ischemic stroke or the hemorrhagic infarction associated with cerebral venous sinus thrombosis [64]. The higher incidence of ICH in COVID-19 patients compared to non-COVID-19 patients [66, 95] is a serious issue. It could be related to a more aggressive treatment with anticoagulation due to a state of hypercoagulability seen in these patients. This condition represents a clinical challenge, obliging closer monitoring of coagulation and control of blood pressure.

Since an analysis on cerebral venous thrombosis in association with COVID-19 identified 57 cases among hospitalized SARS-CoV-2 patients (0.08%), it was suggested a higher occurrence of this serious neurovascular disorder in these infected patients compared to the general population [91]. Cerebral venous sinus thrombosis (CVT) more frequently involves multiple venous vessels. In the retrospective study of Baldini et al. [91], the transverse sinus was most frequently affected (65%), followed by the sigmoid sinus (47%), the superior sagittal sinus (44%), and the straight sinus (21%). The deep venous system was found in 37% of cases, whereas thrombosis in cortical veins was detected in 21% of cases, and hemorrhagic lesions in 42% of cases. A recent study on CVT in COVID-19 found a wide variability of the onset time between the start of COVID-19 clinical presentation and appearance of this complication (from 3 days to 4 months, mean 7–14 days). It could indicate that the pathogenesis of this prothrombotic disease is linked to several factors, such as endothelial damage, altered blood flow pattern, hypercoagulable state, and hyperinflammation. About symptomatology, it varies from alteration of consciousness, to headache, visual symptoms, and focal deficit, such as seizures, hemiparesis, and aphasia. Radiological findings are characterized in most cases by hemorrhagic venous infarcts. The outcome is bad in about one-third of patients [66].

Finally, in some cases, arterial dissection involving extracranial vessels and carotid artery was described. It suggests that SARS-CoV-2 could damage endothelial cells causing the dissection [96, 97].

In the context of COVID-19-associated neurovascular complications, the imaging investigation can offer interesting findings that can help in the differential diagnosis of these CNS manifestations. Lapadopulos et al. [75] offered a detailed analysis. In their study, acute ischemic stroke was the most common neuroimaging finding, with a higher incidence of large vessel occlusion—even in the younger patients—and hemorrhagic transformations; moreover, rare localizations, such as splenium of the corpus callosum, were occasionally described. Again, in a higher number of patients, hemorrhagic stroke showed nontypical locations such as cortical, cortical-subcortical, and lobar locations. These atypical locations lead to some uncertainty on the pathophysiologic mechanisms of ICH. The lesions can be produced by endothelial injury associated with anticoagulation treatment or be the expression of altered regulation of arterial pressure with cerebral hemorrhage. Cerebral microbleeds are another imaging aspect in COVID-19 patients. These lesions are found in atypical locations, such as corpus callosum and juxtacortical white matter; they could be directly related to COVID-19 infection or expression of delayed post-hypoxic leukoencephalopathy. The few cases of cerebral venous thrombosis show the usual pattern with the involvement of deep and superficial veins and sinuses but, in COVID-19 patients, no typical pattern was found. Cases of PRES showed a typical pattern of signal hyperintensities in FLAIR images in occipital, posterior temporal lobes, and the cerebellar hemispheres; in some cases, a hemorrhagic transformation with petechial lesions at the SWI—an MRI sequence that is exquisitely sensitive to venous blood, hemorrhage, and iron storage—was found.

Clinical relevance and outcomes of neurovascular manifestations are a matter of pivotal importance. Tan et al. [84] demonstrated that when occurred in COVID-19 patients, the stroke severity—measured through the NIHSS—was higher than non-COVID-19 patients. These results were confirmed in a study from New York, comparing COVID-19 patients with historical stroke controls. The authors proved a higher NIHSS score in the cohort of COVID-19 patients [90]. Furthermore, in a single-center retrospective analysis from Spain, Hernandez-fernandez et al. [87]

obtained the same significant results (median NIHSS 16 versus 3, $p = 0.006$). Again, in another observational investigation, 67.4% of stroke cases presented with non-focal deficit such as altered mental status ranging from confusion to coma, seizures, generalized weakness, falls, and dizziness, and in the 47.7% of cases, the onset occurred during the hospitalization for COVID-19 [98]. COVID-19 patients could be particularly prone to large vessel occlusion (e.g., internal carotid artery and basilar artery), multi-territory involvement, and uncommonly affected vessels [82, 84]. In the Mendes' et al. [88] study on older patients, the most frequent clinical presentation was an altered consciousness and/or delirium (81.8% of cases), while, in 45.5% of patients, a focal deficit was detected on CT or MRI. In this study a large vessel occlusion was found in 22.2% of patients; stroke was mainly limited to one side (55.5% right, 33.3% left), while the middle cerebral artery territory was affected in 55.5% of cases, followed by the posterior cerebral artery 33.3%, and vertebrobasilar territories 22.2%; in two cases, multiple territories were affected. Similar results were found in another study with a high incidence of large vessel occlusion (58.8%) and unexpectedly high frequency of location in the vertebrobasilar territory (35.5%) [87]. In an analysis on cerebral venous thrombosis, the clinical and neurological features varied from an isolated headache (only in one case) to an altered mental status (the most common sign, 60.5%), to focal deficits–from hemiparesis to aphasia, according to the location of thrombosis—and seizures (27.8%), ranging from focal to status epilepticus [91]. In another international study, 174 consecutive hospitalized COVID-19 patients with ischemic stroke from 16 countries were submitted to a 1:1 propensity score matching analysis with non-COVID-19 patients of Acute Stroke Registry and Analysis of Lausanne Registry. The main stroke symptoms were motor deficits (67.8%), dysarthria (46%), and changes in sensitivity (42%); the median NIHSS was higher in patients with COVID-19 (10 vs. 6, $p = 0.03$) [99].

The outcome reported in the literature is variable, depending on the severity of the underlying cardiorespiratory conditions, the age, and comorbidities of the patients, and the kind of cerebrovascular complication. Katz et al. [98] found in-hospital mortality of 29%, whereas in an Italian case series ($n = 6$) the mortality was 83% with severe neurological sequelae in the survivor (modified Rankin scale, mRS = 4) [100]. In another retrospective study, the outcome of confirmed and suspected COVID-19 was poorer for confirmed or suspected COVID-19 compared to non-COVID-19 patients (adjusted odds ratios, 2.05 [95% CI: 1.12–3.76] and 3.56 [95% CI: 1.15–11.05], respectively [101]. In the Ntaios' study, the mortality was 27.6%; while among the survivors 51% had severe disability at discharge. In the propensity score-matched population, patients with COVID-19 had a higher risk for severe disability (median mRS 4 vs. 2, $p < 0.001$), and death compared with patients without COVID-19 [99]. Another single-center retrospective analysis confirmed a high mortality (34.8%), and showed an unfavorable functional prognosis during the hospital period in 73.9% of patients (17/23 modified Rankin scale, mRS 4–6), with age as the main predictive variable (OR = 1.5; 95% CI: 1.012–2.225; $p = 0.043$) [87]. These results were also confirmed in two systematic reviews that reported a mortality of 38% and 31.5%, respectively [65, 84].

The impact of COVID-19 pandemic on acute stroke care represents one of the most important concerns. The fear of patients being infected when in the hospital could postpone the call to the emergency medical service. Moreover, the burden of work of the prehospital emergency system could further delay the arrival in the hospital. The workload in a crowded emergency department, the time needed to confirm or exclude the infection and to implement the personal and environmental measures of infection prevention, could further delay the definitive treatment. Furthermore, the redeployment of the stroke unit's personnel to face the needing in the emergency and critical care units reduce the capability to respond timely to the needs of acute stroke patients (Fig. 2.3).

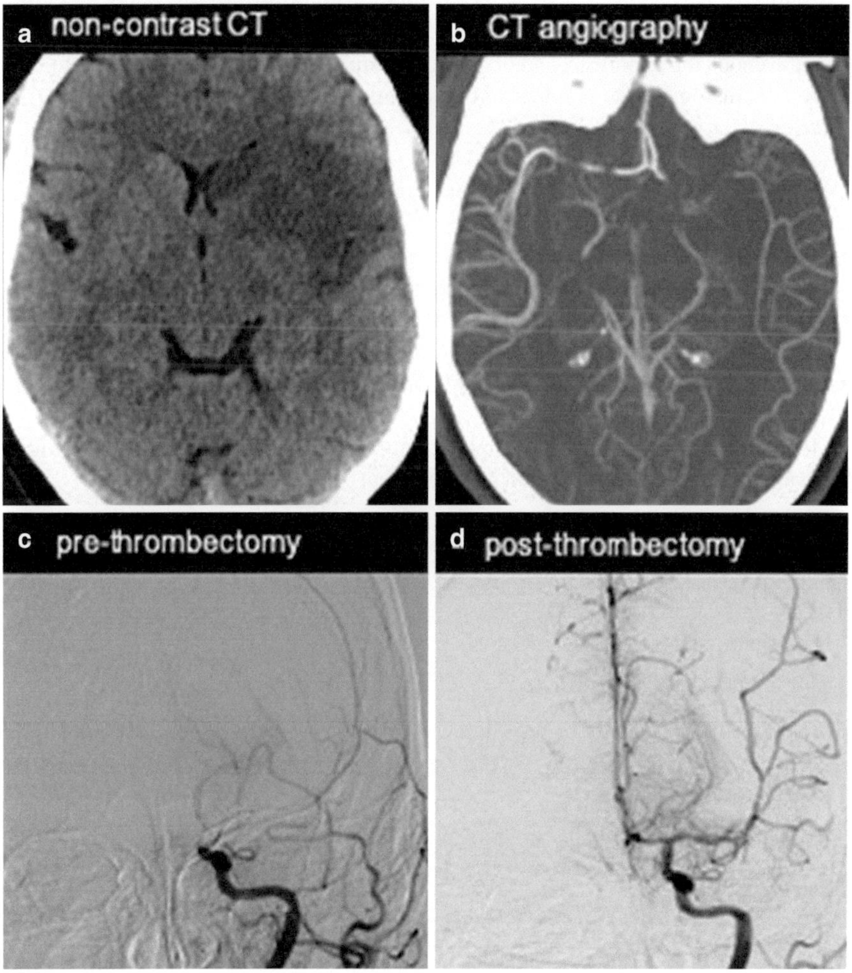

Fig. 2.3 Ischemic stroke treatment. (**a**, **b**) Non-contrast and contrast CT showing acute infarct in the left middle cerebral artery territory. (**c**, **d**) Catheter angiogram before and after revascularization with mechanical thrombectomy. From Agarwall A, et al. Emergency Radiology 2020(27);747–754 with permission

In a retrospective multi-center cohort study on 550 acute stroke patients admitted to seven stroke centers in Madrid, a significant global reduction of stroke admission and secondary transfer from other hospitals was found. Furthermore, significant differences of the time from stroke onset and hospital arrival and delay in median door-to-puncture time were also found [101]. A study from China has demonstrated a drop in hospital admission of 40% compared to the same period of 2019, and a drop in the number of thrombolysis and thrombectomy of 26.7% and 25.3%, respectively. The authors have ascribed these results to many factors, such as the reduced stroke awareness of the patients and their families, an insufficient ambulance resource, the length of the screening process for suspected infected patients, and insufficient stroke medical staff [102]. The German society of neurology confirmed these results, reporting for some Nations a reduction of 40%–50% of hospitalized stroke patients, of 25–41% of intravenous thrombolysis, and of 33% of thrombectomy [36].

In conclusion, stroke is a fearful complication in COVID-19 patients [99–102]. In brief:

- Several risk factors, as age, male sex, history of hypertension, diabetes, and cardiovascular disease were described.
- Some features of COVID-19 disease, such as hyperinflammation and prothrombotic state, can predispose to ischemic and hemorrhagic stroke.
- The incidence of this complication is variable but is higher in most severe patients contributing to a poor outcome.
- The clinical presentation can vary from an altered level of consciousness to focal signs.
- It can be a very early or late complication, compelling the clinician to a thorough evaluation for timely detection and treatment.

Practical Therapeutic Suggestions

The stroke teams should continue treating stroke patients as appropriate with complete adherence to guidelines, adapting the hospital stroke fast-track to the COVID-19 pandemic requirements. To overcome the obstacles in this context and improve assistance, it was suggested [102]:

1. To maintain the stroke awareness programs for the population.
2. To establish a hospital fast-track for COVID-19 screening, integrating the chest CT scan with neck and head CT angiogram for all potential stroke patients.
3. A rapid laboratory test for the SARS-CoV-2 should be prioritized for patients with stroke.
4. The initiation of stroke therapy should not be hindered by the screening process.
5. A specialist of infectious disease should be involved early to allow proper protection of the staff and minimizing delays in the fast-track.

Other strategies are aimed at improving the long-term sequelae. Physical and occupational therapy and rehabilitation planning should be continued during the pandemic, using alternative modalities, such as self-exercise [86].

2.4.6 Meningitis and Encephalitis

Many viruses can cause acute inflammation of the brain and/or the meninges. They include Herpes simplex virus (HSV), Varicella zoster virus (VZV), cytomegalovirus (CMV), influenza virus, and many other respiratory viruses, such as other members of the coronavirus family, like SARS-CoV and MERS-CoV. While it was postulated that also SARS-CoV-2 could potentially cause meningoencephalitis by direct invasion of cerebral tissue [26, 93], only in some cases the virus has been detected in cerebral tissue or in the CSF. The potential mechanisms could be multiple, not only related to direct damage of the virus, but also secondary to the cerebral inflammatory state or immune-mediated response [27].

The first case was described in a 24-year-old patient who, after 9 days from the first respiratory symptoms, showed disturbances of consciousness up to coma (Glasgow Coma Score, GCS 6), generalized seizures, neck stiffness, and laboratory findings showing an increase of neutrophil and a relatively decreased lymphocytes count with increased C-reactive protein (CRP). A brain MRI was performed and DWI showed hyperintensity along the wall of the inferior horn of the right lateral ventricle while FLAIR images demonstrated hyperintense signal changes in the right mesial temporal lobe and hippocampus with slight hippocampal atrophy, contrast-enhanced imaging showed no definite dural enhancement. A lumbar puncture was performed and a clear CSF fluid with a cell count of 12/ml (10 mononuclear and 2 polymorphonuclear cells without red blood cells) was found. The real-time polymerase chain reaction (RT-PCR) test for SARS-CoV-2 detected the virus into the CSF. The clinical, imaging, and laboratory picture allowed diagnosis of right lateral ventriculitis due to SARS-CoV-2 invasion [103]. In another case, a 72-year-old man showed tremor, ataxia, dysarthria, and upper-limb dysmetria with spontaneous diffuse myoclonus 17 days after the onset of SARS-CoV-2 infection. The EEG showed symmetric diffuse background slowing, reactive to stimulation, without interictal paroxysm. Moreover, brain MRI with contrast showed no lesions and the CSF examination indicated a normal cell count, a mildly elevated protein level (49 mg/dL), and a negative RT-PCR test. On the other hand, the immunologic study on serum and CSF revealed high titers of IgG autoantibodies directed against the nuclei of Purkinje cells, striatal neurons, and hippocampal neurons. Again, brain ^{18}F-fluorodeoxyglucose (^{18}F-FDG) positron emission tomography (PET) indicated diffuse cortical hypometabolism as well as putaminal and cerebellum hypermetabolism. These findings allowed the diagnosis of autoimmune encephalitis [104].

Various literature reviews report other potential cases of COVID-19-associated encephalitis. In these cases, clinical signs varied from agitation, disorientation, meningeal rigidity, and photophobia to hallucinations, reduced level of consciousness, and focal status epilepticus. When performed, lumbar puncture showed normal CSF or a lymphocytic pleocytosis and elevated protein level; in some cases, the RT-PCR test for SARS-CoV-2 detected the virus in CSF. Furthermore, EEG studies showed generalized slowing or focal signs and the neuroimaging study highlighted several data, although generally not very indicative of damage. In particular, brain CT was reported normal in the majority of cases or showed areas of hypoattenuation, and MRI studies were normal in some reports, while cortical hyperintensities with sulcal effacement in some areas of the brain were rarely found [27, 85, 93].

In a retrospective observational study on 222 hospitalized COVID-19 patients with neurologic manifestations, encephalitis was defined as an altered mental status lasting more than 24 hours along with the following criteria:

- WBC in CSF < 5/mm^3; or
- presence of a compatible acute lesion on brain MRI; and
- acute meningitis defined as a meningeal syndrome (head stiffness, headache, fever)

Encephalitis was detected in 9.5% of the patients (median age 67 years). Half of these exhibited a focal neurologic deficit in addition to altered mental status, with predominant cerebellar ataxia and pyramidal syndrome. Just over a quarter of patients had movement disorders, mostly tremor and myoclonus, whereas brain MRI was abnormal in two-thirds of patients with imaging compatible with encephalitis and CSF examination demonstrated lymphocytic pleocytosis, with WBC count from 6 to 77/mm^3, in two-thirds of patients. Of note, the SARS-CoV-2 PCR test in CSF was positive in only two patients, whereas EEG was abnormal in 93.3% of patients. The authors reported a mortality rate of 4.8% [37]. Interestingly, other authors reported a lower prevalence of acute meningitis and/or encephalitis (0.5%) [25].

In order to identify specific clinical characteristics of encephalitis/meningitis associated with COVID-19, a recent literature review investigated on 32 encephalitis/meningitis. Neurologic symptoms appeared after 1 week from the onset of COVID-19 symptomatology (range 1–21 days). The most common symptoms were consciousness disturbances (59.3%), seizure (21.8%), delirium (18.7%), and headache (18.7%). Four patients were positive to RT-PCR for SARS-CoV2 in CSF, one in postoperative brain tissue and one was positive for SARS-CoV2 antibodies in CSF. Neuroimaging showed mainly damage at the level of the temporal lobe (15%), frontal lobe (9%), corpus callosum (9%), white matter (12%), cervical spine cord (12%), thalami (9%), and cortex (6%). Notably, 30% of patients were submitted to electroencephalography (EEG) studies to assess unexplained consciousness disturbances, myoclonus, seizure, headache, and dysarthria; in 80% of cases, EEG showed diffuse slow wave, and in 20% focal epileptic wave [105].

A rare form of encephalitis seen during COVID-19 is the acute necrotizing encephalitis (ANE). Usually, it develops by various viral infections, such as influenza A and B, herpesvirus, varicella, and rotavirus, and affects predominantly children [68]. Etiology seems related to the systemic cytokine storm that alters BBB permeability without vessel disruption, viral invasion, and para-infectious demyelination [69]. The clinical picture is fulminant and not specific and can be characterized, after a prodromal stage, by a disturbance of consciousness, seizures, focal deficits accompanied with decerebrate and decorticate posture, followed, in the recovery stage, by neurological sequelae [67]. The CT findings are characterized by a multifocal symmetric distribution of petechial hemorrhage and necrosis of gray and white matter distributed to cerebral white matter, thalami, with a characteristic bilateral involvement, brainstem and cerebellum; MRI shows a hyperintense signal with internal hemorrhage [67, 68]. The first case of ANE during COVID-19 was described, in the US, in a female COVID-19 patient with a history of cough, fever, as well as typical mental status alterations, and CT, and RMI findings [69]. In another case, the clinical picture was characterized by stupor and myoclonus that occurred late-onset from the respiratory symptoms. The neurological conditions worsened until the rapid development of a coma. Nevertheless, there were no signs of a hyperinflammatory state. Of note, CT and MRI findings were typical for ANE and the RT-PCR test for SARS-CoV-2 in CSF confirmed the diagnosis of COVID-19-associated ANE [70]. In another case, a 72-year-old man, positive for SARS-CoV-2 (RT-PCR test), with agitation/delirium, developed severe respiratory distress that required intubation and mechanical ventilation. At the resolution of respiratory problems, the level of consciousness remained low and reduced strength of the limbs was detected; an MRI study revealed acute lacunar infarcts in the right frontal deep white matter and a few small FLAIR hyperintense foci in the bilateral periventricular white matter. There was no significant stenosis or occlusion of the intracranial arteries. The SWI further demonstrated multiple microhemorrhages which were diffusely distributed in the bilateral cortical-juxtacortical regions, deep white matter, basal ganglia, corpus callosum, brainstem, and cerebellum. Again, investigations on CSF were negative for inflammatory meningoencephalitis and SARS-CoV-2. After discharge, the patient's neurological conditions remained severely compromised with a low GCS. It was postulated that endotheliitis with thrombotic microangiopathy can represent the underlying mechanism of these findings (cerebral microbleeds and leukoencephalopathy). They also concluded that other mechanisms, such as excessive inflammation and prolonged hypoxemic respiratory failure, cannot be excluded [71].

The acute disseminated encephalomyelitis (ADEM) is another rare autoimmune disease of the CNS that can occur after a viral infection, mainly affecting children; nevertheless, in COVID-19, the few case reports of ADEM regarded patients in middle to old age. The clinical symptoms vary from focal neurological deficits (optic neuritis, severe paresis) to a subacute encephalopathic syndrome. The therapy includes high-dose steroids and intravenous immunoglobulins [36]. The first case described of COVID-19-related ADEM was a 40-year-old female who after 11 days from the onset of headache and myalgia developed fever, tachypnea, and mild hypoxemia. She was alert and sluggishly followed commands; additionally, she showed dysarthria, expressive aphasia, dysphagia, and facial weakness; there was no meningismus, and the patient showed a mild bilateral decrease of strength with preserved deep tendon reflex. The molecular test for SARS-CoV-2 was positive.

The CSF analysis revealed normal cells, proteins, and glucose. Furthermore, the head CT showed multiple areas of patchy hypoattenuation, and the MRI found areas of increased FLAIR and T2 signal consistent with demyelination the in frontoparietal white matter of both hemispheres, anterior temporal lobes, basal ganglia, external capsule, and thalami [106]. Other rare cases were described. A 71-year-old man showed fatigue and dyspnea rapidly developing in progressive cardiorespiratory failure, postoperatively after elective cardiac surgery. The molecular test for SARS-CoV-2 was positive and the clinical conditions further worsened until requiring ICU admission. The clinical picture was suggestive of a fatal highly inflammatory state. The autopsy showed a range of neuropathological lesions, with vascular and demyelinating etiologies. They comprised hemorrhagic white matter lesions in the cerebral hemispheres with surrounding axonal injury and macrophages, scattered clusters of macrophages in subcortical white matter with associated axonal injury, focal microscopic areas of necrosis with central loss of white matter and marked axonal injury, and perivascular ADEM-like appearance [33]. Another case of ADEM was seen in a 51 years old man presenting with symptoms of COVID-19 (fever, nausea, dyspnea, and hypoxia). The chest Rx revealed bilateral patchy opacifications; the SARS-CoV-2 RT-PCR from a nasopharyngeal swab was positive. The patient was intubated and admitted to ICU where he received mechanical ventilation under sedation for 18 days; afterward, he was transferred to another facility where the sedation was stopped for a neurological evaluation. The exam showed a GCS = 3, pupils equal, round, and reactive to light, corneal responses intact and the left oculocephalic response impaired; the muscles were bilaterally flaccid, and no movements were noted spontaneously or in response to pain; deep tendon reflexes were depressed and plantar responses were mute. The brain MRI highlighted scattered hyperintense lesions on FLAIR imaging in deep hemispheric and juxtacortical white matter. These lesions were hyperintense on DWI; among these lesions, a minority showed subtle restricted diffusion on the apparent diffusion coefficient; a FLAIR hyperintensity in the left frontal juxtacortical white matter showed mild enhancement with gadolinium contrast. A small amount of intraventricular hemorrhage was found in both lateral ventricles. The CSF study demonstrated xanthochromia, proteins (62 mg/dl), and glucose (56 mg/dl). SARS-CoV-2 was not detected in the CSF. High-dose steroids and intravenous immunoglobulins were prescribed and, in 1 week, the patient showed a progressive improvement of clinical condition, becoming conscious and able to speak [72].

A variant of the ADEM, the acute hemorrhagic leukoencephalomyelitis (AHLE), was found in a 33-year-old male with chronic renal disease and hypertension. The patient showed an acute onset of the symptoms with progressive weakness of both upper and lower limbs and reduced consciousness of recent onset. In the emergency department, the patient had an episode of generalized tonic-clonic seizures, treated with antiepileptic drugs. The clinical evaluation showed a GCS of 7, no neck rigidity, and deep tendon reflexes absent in all four limbs with bilateral extensor plantar response. The MRI study revealed symmetrical FLAIR hyperintensities involving bilateral subcortical frontoparietal lobes, splenium of the corpus callosum, medulla, and cervical cord with petechial hemorrhages and evidence of diffusion restriction involving splenium of corpus callosum. Again, the chest X-ray showed bilateral opacities and the EEG was suggestive of a diffuse slowing with no epileptiform discharges. The study of CSF demonstrated normal protein, glucose, and cellular count, whereas hematologic exams showed elevated inflammatory indices and the RT-PCR test for SARS-CoV-2 from the nasopharyngeal swab was positive. The patient was admitted to the ICU. A final diagnosis of AHLE was made and steroid therapy was started. After as few days, the clinical conditions improved and the patient became conscious and responsive to the command. Finally, the motor deficit improved in upper and lower limbs. Unfortunately, the cardiorespiratory conditions worsened and the patient died [73].

MRI studies could help in differential diagnosis of these forms of acute encephalitis. In fact, ADEM is characterized by multiple, asymmetric, poorly marginated lesions, smaller in size, with less severe edema and additional spinal cord involvement, without hemorrhage and enhancement. ANE shows characteristic symmetric signal changes with thalamic involvement and additional lesions at the level of the brainstem, cerebral white matter, and cerebellum. AHLE demonstrates multifocal, with variable size, poorly defined white matter lesions involving both cerebral hemispheres, mainly in parietal and occipital lobes, particularly in subcortical and deep white matter, with characteristic asymmetric distribution, and affecting less frequently also brainstem, cerebellar peduncle, and deep grey matter [74].

In conclusion, due to the lack of clear definitions and the multiform clinical and histopathological features, it is difficult to establish the relationship between SARS-CoV-2 infection and meningoencephalitis. Even in the cases where the virus was detected in brain tissue and/or in CSF, the etiopathogenesis could be variable and depending on other causes, such as ischemic/hypoxic encephalopathy or multiorgan failure, especially in most severe patients.

Practical Therapeutic Suggestions

The suggested treatment consists of supporting vital functions to prevent further damage. In the case of negative pathogen diagnostics and persistence of symptoms, the use of corticosteroids in high doses (e.g., methylprednisolone 1 g/day for 3–5 days) is advised [36].

2.4.7 Acute Myelitis

The first case of myelitis was described in China by Zhao et al. [76]. A 66-year-old male, with a 5-day history of fever and fatigue, was admitted to the hospital where a nasopharyngeal swab resulted positive for RT-PCR SARS-CoV-2. After an episode of hyperthermia, the patient developed weakness in both lower limbs with urinary and bowel incontinence, up to flaccid lower-extremity paralysis. Neurologic examination showed a decreased strength in the arms with normal bilateral reflexes in upper extremities, and flaccid paralysis in the legs with bilateral hyporeflexia but without pathologic reflexes. The sensation was intact in the arms but globally impaired in both legs with a T10 sensory level, with paresthesia and numbness below the level. The tendon reflexes of the lower limbs were decreased. Inflammatory laboratory tests were increased with high values of ferritin, leucocytes, CRP, accompanied by lymphopenia. The brain CT revealed basal ganglia and paraventricular lacunar infarctions, while MRI of spinal cord was not performed. The patient was treated with antivirals, antibiotics, steroids, immunoglobulins, and supportive therapy. His muscle strength showed a good recovery in both the upper limbs, and only a limited recovery in the lower limbs.

Other case reports were reported in the literature. A 32-year-old man presented with sudden paraplegia and urinary retention after a 2-day history of flu-like symptoms. There was no sensory deficit nor upper limbs weakness or back pain. Neurological examination revealed normal muscle tone in the upper limbs, and hypotonia in both lower limbs, with complete paralysis. There was also trunk weakness without the involvement of the neck muscles. An MRI revealed extensive diffuse hyperintense signal involving predominantly the grey matter of the cervical, dorsal, and lumbar regions of the spinal cord, with mild enlargement and swelling of the cervical cord; DWI and apparent diffusion coefficient (ADC) revealed areas of restricted diffusion. A treatment with pulse dose of intravenous methylprednisolone, acyclovir, and enoxaparin was initiated, and after 5 days a marked improvement was noted [77]. Another patient developed bladder dysfunction and progressive weakness of the lower limbs after 8 days from the first symptoms of SARS-CoV-2 infection. The neurological examination showed hypesthesia below the T9 level and a moderate spastic paraparesis with Babinski's sign positive bilaterally. The first MRI revealed T2 signal hyperintensity of the thoracic spinal cord at T9 level suggestive of acute transverse myelitis; CSF analysis was abnormal with lymphocytic pleocytosis and elevated protein level, but SARS-CoV-2 RT-PCR and oligoclonal bands were negative. Methylprednisolone was started and the patient improved rapidly [78].

Clinical laboratory and imaging findings of 18 cases of myelitis during COVID-19 pandemic were reviewed [79]. The mean time from the first symptoms of the disease and the onset of myelitis was 10.3 ± 7.8 days. Motor symptoms were present in 88.9% of cases with different degrees of paresis, and complete quadri- or paraplegia in one-third of patients. A sensitive impairment was present in 77.7% of cases, and sphincter dysfunction in 88.8%. The most common syndrome was transverse myelitis (77.7%), followed by partial transverse myelitis (11.1%), Brown Sequard syndrome (5.5%), and dorsal columns syndrome (5.5%). Myelitis was associated with few cases with encephalitis, optic neuritis, or GBS. CSF showed mild pleocytosis and moderate elevation of proteins in most of the patients. At MRI about one-third of patients showed brain abnormalities, 88.2% spinal cord abnormalities, with a prevalent localization in cervico-thoracic level (50%) and a mean lesion length of 6 segments [79]. Another study on neuroimaging features confirmed isolated or multifocal hyperintense lesions on STIR or T2-weighted MRI images in the cervical and thoracic cord, in some cases accompanied by tissue edema. The presence of cytotoxic edema was confirmed by the restricted diffusion on diffusion-weighted imaging and apparent diffusion coefficient sequences [75].

In the review of Rodríguez de Antonio et al. [79] the suggested pathological mechanisms were linked to cytokines released by inflammatory storms or para-infectious immune mediated, as confirmed by the MRI findings and the response to corticosteroids and intravenous IG (IVIG) therapy [79]. Interestingly, a complete/moderate recovery was observed in one-third of cases, and mild improvement in half of the patients [79].

Practical Therapeutic Suggestions

- The most common treatment consists of corticosteroids (e.g., methylprednisolone 1 g/day for 3–5 days).
- Other treatments are IVIG (400 mg/kg/day for 5 days), and plasma-exchange for 2–7 sessions (frequently in combination with corticosteroids).

2.5 PNS Manifestations

This group encompasses hypo/anosmia and dysgeusia/ageusia alterations, GBS, and pain (Table 2.2). Injuries to the cranial nerves also fall into this group; they are described in terms of case reports or case series and mainly concern ophthalmoparesis, or facial nerve palsy [114].

Table 2.2 PNS manifestations of COVID-19

Clinical manifestation [Ref.]	Features	Occurrence	Pathogenesis
Smell and taste impairment [75, 107]	Hypo/anosmia, parosmia, olfactory hallucinations, fluctuating hyposmia dysgeusia/ageusia	5.6–85.6%	Damage of the cells of the olfactory epithelium due to direct viral action or cytokine storm
Guillain-Barré syndrome [108]	Ascending flaccid paralysis with areflexia/hyporeflexia, and sensory deficits	0.15‰ (increased in demyelinating subtypes)	Immune mediated: Molecular mimicry between viral proteins and proteins on peripheral nerves leading to autoantibody-mediated damage to myelin or axons. Massive release of cytokines and macrophage activation during the cytokine storm
Pain [109–113]	Headache, muscle/joint pain, chest, and abdominal pain	6–44%	Multifactorial: Proinflammatory cytokines, direct/indirect viral damage
Cranial nerve injuries [114]	Ophthalmoparesis, or facial nerve palsy (unilaterally or bilaterally)	Case reports/series	Direct viral damage; ischemia of *vasa nervorum*; demyelination induced by an inflammatory process

2.5.1 Hypo/Anosmia and Dysgeusia/Ageusia

The prevalence of smell and taste impairment varies widely in the literature, ranging from 5.6% to 88% for taste impairment and from 5.1% to 98% for smell impairment. These differences depend on the severity of the disease, differences in population food habit, potential mutations of the virus, underestimation of the olfactory manifestation, study design, and method of testing [26, 114–116]. For example, olfactory dysfunction had a high incidence in European and American countries compared to the Chinese population [115].

Anosmia or ageusia may be the sole presenting symptom in approximately 3% of patients [14, 114]. It is still uncertain whether the taste and smell alterations are due to inflammation of the nasal tract or damage to the sensory neurons in the olfactory bulb [116]. About the clinical relevance and outcomes, complete recovery was reported in the majority of patients [28, 116]. Nevertheless, a recent observational study from 18 European hospitals proved that when patients were carefully evaluated with objective olfactory tests, about 15% of those with anosmia still showed deficiency at 60 days, and 4.7% had not recovered olfaction at 6 months [117]. It was also demonstrated that the prevalence of olfactory dysfunction was significantly higher in mild forms (85.9%) compared with moderate-to-critical forms (4.5–6.9%; $p = 0.001$) and that the mean duration was 21.6 ± 17.9 days [117]. Another study from the same group ($n = 2579$) confirmed the higher prevalence of olfactory dysfunction (73.7%) and gustatory dysfunction (46.8%), with higher prevalence in mild forms of COVID-19, and in females and diabetic patients [118].

In a retrospective observational study on 646 confirmed COVID-19 patients, of whom 88 required hospitalization, smell and taste impairment were reported in 37.9% and 36.8% of cases, respectively. Among patients with smell impairment, 65.3% had complete anosmia, 26.6% parosmia, 10.9% olfactory hallucinations, and 24.9% fluctuating hyposmia. Patients with taste impairment reported complete ageusia in 63.2%; moreover, 79.4% had an altered taste of sweetness, 79.9% altered taste of saltiness, 71.4% altered acid taste, and 66% altered taste of bitterness. The majority of the patients reported combined smell and taste impairment. The median time from the disease onset to the development of smell and taste impairment was 2–3 days. Only 38.4% of patients reported concomitant nasal obstruction. A complete recovery was observed in 72.1% cases of smell impairment and 76.8% of taste impairment [38].

In a large systematic review and meta-analysis on 32,142 COVID-19 patients from 107 studies, the prevalence of anosmia was 38.2% (95% CI: 36.5%, 47.2%), while the prevalence of dysgeusia was 36.6% (95% CI: 35.2%, 45.2%) [107].

About the pathogenesis of smell and taste impairment, several mechanisms have been invoked to explain the emergence of this symptomatology. The presence of ACE2 receptors in the cells of the olfactory epithelium, with the function of supporting the olfactory neurons, could suggest a direct viral damage of these cells leading to a dysfunction of the olfactory neurons. Another possible mechanism is the olfactory epithelium dysfunction caused by the proinflammatory cytokines during the acute phase of the disease. The hypothesized mechanisms of direct damage of the olfactory sensory neurons or of the olfactory center via axonal transport seem less possible [107].

Since in most cases anosmia is typically not accompanied by nasal congestion and the onset in the majority of cases is sudden, it was proposed that every patient presenting with isolated anosmia should be screened for SARS-CoV-2, especially in the pandemic contest [26, 28]. Furthermore, it was proposed that, in addition to the current symptom criteria used to trigger quarantine, any adult with anosmia but no other symptoms should self-isolate for seven days [19].

The guidelines of the German Society of Neurology [36] stated that:

1. During the pandemic, a suddenly appearing olfactory disorder (anosmia) during free nasal breathing is very likely an expression of SARS-CoV-2 infection.
2. Olfactory disturbances can precede other disease symptoms and are therefore epidemiologically relevant (early identification of new "hot spots").
3. The olfactory disorder in COVID-19 seems to be mostly temporary. Whether or not complete restitution is regularly achieved cannot yet be conclusively assessed.
4. When the olfactory function does not return to normal within 3–4 weeks, neurological and ENT evaluation with further diagnostics is recommended.

Practical Therapeutic Suggestions

Long-term olfactory problems can be managed through:

- Olfactory training (by combining visual imagery with the stimulation of an isolated scent). Eventually combined with:
  - Neuroprotective agents (e.g., palmitoylethanolamide (PEA) plus scutellaria baicalensis root extract)
  - Topic or oral steroids

2.5.2 Guillain-Barré Syndrome and Variants

It is an acute immune-mediated polyradiculoneuropathy affecting motor, sensory, and autonomic nerves. The disease presents with various neurological manifestations; the most common is an ascending flaccid paralysis with areflexia/hyporeflexia, and sensory deficits that spread over days to weeks (acute inflammatory demyelinating polyneuropathy, AIDP). Nevertheless, GBS can often include cranial nerves impairment, with the involvement of the facial nerve being the most common. Again, in the most severe cases, GBS could rapidly progress to respiratory failure. Classically, the CSF study reveals an albuminocytologic dissociation [26, 119]. It can develop after gastrointestinal and respiratory infections. Potential trigger factors could be viruses such as Zika virus, Epstein–Barr virus, and influenza virus, and bacteria such as Campylobacter jejuni, and Mycoplasma pneumoniae as well as other factors including cancer diseases, anticancer drugs, vaccinations, and surgery.

Interestingly, neuromuscular disorders were reported in patients affected by different coronaviruses, mostly the MERS-CoV [120].

Classically, the symptomatology appears after a certain period of time from the infection and the appearance of the neurological symptoms [28]. Some variants of GBS were described [119]. They include:

- Acute inflammatory demyelinating polyradiculoneuropathy (AIDP)
- Acute motor axonal neuropathy (AMAN)
- Acute motor and sensory axonal neuropathy (AMSAN)
- Miller Fisher Syndrome (MFS)
- Paraparetic GBS
- Pharyngeal-cervical-brachial weakness
- Bilateral facial palsy with paresthesia (BFP)
- Bickerstaff brainstem encephalitis (BBE)
- Polyneuritis cranialis or GBS-MFS overlap (PNC)
- Acute autonomic neuropathy

Interestingly, the AIDP and AMAN variants were documented after SARS-CoV infections while cases of AIDP, AMAN, and BBE were reported in MERS-CoV disease [26].

First reports of the association of GBS with SARS-CoV-19 were described in China [121] and Iran [122]. In the first case, a 61-year-old woman presented to the hospital with acute severe symmetric weakness in both legs and areflexia in both legs and feet. The symptoms worsened within a few days with muscle strength grade 4/5 in both arms and hands and 3/5 in both legs and feet; the sensation to light touch and pinprick was decreased distally. Laboratory findings showed lymphocytopenia and thrombocytopenia while CSF showed normal cell counts and increased protein level. On day 5, the nerve conduction study showed delayed distal latencies and absent F waves in the early course, supporting demyelinating neuropathy. The patient developed symptoms of COVID-19 (fever, cough with bilateral ground-glass opacities on lung CT scan) only on day 8 of hospital admission and, at that time, oropharyngeal swab resulted positive for SARS-CoV-2. Treatment with IV immunoglobulins and antiviral drugs was started and the patient was discharged with normal muscle strength. As the symptoms of GBS overlapped with those of SARS-CoV-19 the authors recognized in this case a profile of pattern of a para-infectious profile, instead of the classic post-infectious profile of GBS [121]. In the second report, a 65-year-old male patient was admitted to the hospital with symptoms of acute progressive symmetric ascending quadriparesis and bilateral facial paresis starting 5 days before, and 2 weeks after a diagnosis of COVID-19. The muscle strength examination showed weakness in four limbs with a Medical Research Council (MRC) 0–5 scale of 2/5 in proximal, 3/5 in distal of the upper extremities and 1/5 in proximal, 2/5 in distal of the lower extremities. Deep tendon reflexes were generally absent, and there was no spine sensory level, nor meningeal irritation signs. CSF analysis was not performed. Cervical and brain MRI was negative, while electrodiagnostic parameters demonstrated decreased amplitude at compound muscle action potential and no response at sensory nerve action potential; electromyography showed decreased recruitment. The patient was treated with IV immunoglobulins according to the diagnosis of GBS [121].

In a case series from Italy, five patients presented with weakness and paresthesia as their main symptoms. Four of them were immediately positive for COVID-19, whereas 1 turned positive later. All patients developed GBS 5–10 days following COVID-19 symptoms onset. Lower-limb weakness and paresthesia were the main presenting features in four patients, followed by facial weakness, ataxia, and paresthesia in one patient. The CSF was normocellular in all five cases; albuminocytological dissociation was found in three cases. Electrophysiological studies showed reduced compound motor amplitudes and prolonged distal latencies. The overall neurophysiological pattern was considered typical of demyelination in two cases and compatible with an axonal neuropathy in the remaining three cases. Fibrillation potentials were seen by electromyography (EMG) acutely in three patients, and later in a fourth patient. None of the patients had SARS-CoV-2 detected in the CSF (RT-PCR). Antiganglioside antibodies were absent in the three tested patients. Post-gadolinium MRI showed caudal nerve roots enhancement in two patients, facial nerve enhancement in another patient, and no signal changes in two patients. All patients received IV immunoglobulin and one plasma-exchange. After 4 weeks of therapy, two patients were still on ventilator support, two received physical therapy for paraplegia, and another one was discharged and was able to walk independently [123].

Other less common variants of GBS have been reported in patients with COVID-19. MFS presents with acute-onset external ophthalmoplegia and ataxia associated with the loss of tendon reflexes. Gutierrez-Ortiz et al. [124] described two cases. One of these concerned a 50-year-old man with a history of vertical diplopia, and gait instability after a story of fever, cough, headache, malaise, anosmia, and ageusia. The neurological examination showed perioral paresthesia without facial weakness; strength and muscle tone were normal in all extremities, and no sensory deficits were detected. He had a broad-based ataxic gait and absent deep tendon reflexes in both the upper and lower limbs; furthermore, the patient showed right internuclear ophthalmoparesis and right fascicular oculomotor palsy. The laboratory exams indicated lymphopenia, and elevated C-reactive protein. Antibodies to the ganglioside GD1b—commonly associated with severe GBS forms and the requirement of mechanical ventilation—were found. The swab RT-PCR for COVID-19 was positive. The CSF revealed no WBC, protein 80 mg/dl, glucose 62 mg/dl, with normal cytology, and sterile cultures. The viral genome was not detected in the CSF and the head CT scan was normal. The patient was treated with IV immunoglobulins with an improvement of symptoms and he was discharged at home 2 weeks after admission. Another 39-year-old man presented with diplopia 3 days after he had diarrhea, fever, and ageusia. On neurological examination, he showed severe abduction deficits in both eyes, and fixation nystagmus, with the upper gaze more impaired, all consistent with bilateral abducens palsy. All deep tendon reflexes were absent. The neurological examination of limbs, including sensation, was normal. No gait instability or truncal ataxia was observed. The oropharyngeal swab was positive for SARS-CoV-2, CSF analysis showed cell count 2/μl (all monocytes), protein 62 mg/dl, glucose 50 mg/dl, with normal cytology, sterile cultures, and negative serology, including the RT-PCR for COVID-19. The patient was labeled as having a polyneuritis cranialis and treated with acetaminophen; after 2 weeks he had complete recovery of neurological symptoms [124].

Another case of MSF was more recently described by Kajani et al. [125]. A 50-year-old male with a past medical history of obesity, diabetes, and heroin use arrived in the hospital after 4 days of slurred speech and progressive difficulty with swallowing. His nasopharyngeal swab was positive for RT-PCR for COVID-19. The patient presented with palate weakness and nasal voice, bilateral ptosis, and generalized internal and external ophthalmoplegia in all directions. On motor examination, he had normal tone and strength in upper and lower limbs. Reflexes in the patient's upper extremities were absent, and in the lower extremities slight patellar reflexes were found. He had mild dysmetria and dysdiadochokinesia in the upper extremities. Brain CT and MRI were normal. The patient had increasing difficulty protecting his airway and was intubated and ventilated. The descending weakness progressed to his shoulder, proximal upper extremity, and muscles of respiration. CSF analysis showed zero WBC, and a slight increase of proteins, while CSF SARS-CoV-2 PCR was negative. Serum ganglioside antibodies were all negative. Although the patient was treated with IV immunoglobulins, he died due to cardiac complications in a few days.

In a retrospective multi-center registry from France, including COVID-19 patients with neurological manifestations ($n = 222$), GBS was the most common neurologic manifestation (6.8%) following encephalopathy, stroke, and encephalitis. The median age was 59 years, and 66.7% of patients had mild or moderate COVID-19. CSF examinations were performed in 14 patients, demonstrating isolated elevated protein levels in 57.1% of them, ranging from 0.49 to 2.36 g/L. Negative SARS-CoV-2 RT-PCR results were obtained in nine patients tested. Electroneuromyography was performed in 14 patients and was suggestive of demyelination in 92.9% of them. The majority of patients (93.3%) were treated with IV immunoglobulin. Two patients required mechanical ventilation and there was no mortality during the follow-up [37].

On the topic, a systematic review on 52 studies and 73 patients was also published. The authors found that the mean age at onset was 55 ± 17 years (min 11–max 94), there was a significant prevalence of men (68.5% vs. 31.5%), and no prevalence of particular comorbidities was noticed. In 94.5% of patients, GBS manifestations developed after those of COVID-19 (min 2, max 33 days); in the other cases, COVID-19 symptoms were concurrent or occurred 1–8 days after GBS onset. Common clinical manifestations at onset included sensory symptoms (72.2%) alone or in combination with paraparesis or tetraparesis; cranial nerve involvement was less frequent (16.7%). All cases but one showed lower limbs or generalized areflexia, whereas in 37.5% of them, gait ataxia was reported at onset or during the disease course. Ascending weakness evolved into flaccid tetraparesis in 76% of patients and spreading/persistence of sensory symptoms represented the most common clinical evolutions (84.7%). Furthermore, 50% and 23.6% of patients showed, respectively, cranial nerve deficits and dysphagia during the disease course. Of note, 36.1% of patients developed respiratory symptoms up to respiratory failure in some cases. Autonomic disturbances were rare (16.7%). In cases with MFS/MFS-GBS overlap, areflexia (100%), oculomotor disturbances (66.7%), and ataxia (66.7%) were found. The electrophysiological study showed a pattern compatible with a demyelinating polyradiculoneuropathy in 77.4%, axonal damage in 14.5%, and a mixed pattern in 8.1% of patients. The albuminocytological dissociation (cell count less than 5/μl with elevated CSF proteins) was detected in 71.2% of the cases with a median CSF protein of 100 mg/dl (49–317 mg/dl); mild pleocytosis was found in 8.5% of patients. In this series CSF SARS-CoV-2 RNA was undetectable in all tested patients, while the antiganglioside antibodies were positive in 5,7% of patients. The MRI study showed a cranial nerve contrast enhancement (in MFS, and BFP); brainstem leptomeningeal enhancement in two cases of AIDP. About therapy, 85.8% of patients were treated with IV immunoglobulins, 14.2% with plasma-exchange, and 2.8% with steroids [120].

A recent review on 220 cases, confirmed that the onset of syndrome occurred after the onset of the non-neurological symptoms in most of cases, but few cases could occur together or before the other symptomatology. The most common subtype was AIDP (77.6%), followed by AMAN (8.5%) and ASMAN (7.2%) subtypes, and less frequently by MFS (4.6%), PNC (1.3%), and PCB (0.65%) variants. The outcome reported a complete recovery in 22% of patients, partial recovery in 70.8% of subjects, and death in 7.1% of cases. This study offered a further proof about the need to exclude other differential diagnoses, such as critically ill neuromyopathy, toxic neuropathy, and the effects of drugs, and to make an early diagnosis for an appropriate treatment [108].

The pathogenic mechanism of GBS and its variants was reported to the molecular similarity of some virus epitopes with surface neurons' components. In particular, antibodies produced against the pathogen could bind the peripheral nerve components (e.g., antiganglioside antibodies), destroying the neurons. Another possible mechanism is the macrophage activation during the cytokine storm [26]. The typical latency of neurological symptoms observed in most patients, the clinical and biochemical findings, and the improvement after IV immunoglobulins therapy, seems to support the post-infectious immune-mediated mechanism, although the massive release of cytokines in COVID-19 may also have a role in the dysimmune process. In COVID-19 patients, thus, the pathogenic mechanisms seem to reflect the features of the classic post-infective GBS [104]. Nevertheless, patients with prolonged admission in ICU, ventilated in the prone position, treated with neuromuscular blockers and steroids, and suffered from sepsis and multiorgan failure, could develop myopathy and neuropathy leading to an overt ICU-acquired weakness. These complex patients need to enter into a differential diagnosis.

Practical Therapeutic Suggestions
According to the guidelines of the German Society of Neurology [36]:

- A serological test for ganglioside antibodies is suggested (particularly in cases of cranial nerve involvement).
- The therapy should not differ from the usual treatment for GBS.
- The primary use of IV immunoglobulins (0.4 g/kg) is preferred but plasma-exchange is considered equivalent.
- Corticosteroids should be avoided.

2.5.3 Pain

Pain is commonly reported during the SARS-CoV-2 infection [126]. Headache and muscle/joint pain are among the most frequently reported symptoms either in mild and more severe forms. Less frequent reported forms of pain are chest and abdominal pain, eye pain, and sore throat [109]. In a study on the general population in USA, a periodic longitudinal questionnaire was administered to 21,359 subjects regardless of history of COVID-19 infection or test. In this survey various types of pain were described: muscle pain was reported in 53.6% of hospitalized and 71% of non-hospitalized patients, pain between shoulder blades in 47.3% of hospitalized and 62.6% of non-hospitalized patients, pain/burning feeling in lungs in 47.5% of hospitalized and 49.6% of non-hospitalized patients, burning feeling in trachea in 33% of hospitalized and 35.1% of non-hospitalized patients, joint pain in 33% of hospitalized and 43.8% of non-hospitalized patients, ear pain in 10.7% of hospitalized and 21.4% of non-hospitalized patients [80].

Many hypotheses have been proposed to explain the presence of pain during the SARS-CoV-2 infection: the high level of proinflammatory cytokines, the direct or para-infectious immunomediated viral damage of the peripheral nerves, could all lead to the onset of pain during the acute phase of the disease and its subsequent persistence in the chronic phase [110]. Furthermore, neuropathic pain could follow other neurological complications such as stroke, myelitis, and GBS [111]. Finally, patients with chronic pain could experience an exacerbation of the symptomatology due to multiple factors including discontinuation of therapy and psychological burden of the pandemic [111].

Pain is a clinical manifestation of long-COVID. In particular, combined or not with other symptoms such as anxiety and depression, brain fog, fatigue, shortness of breath, and others, osteoarticular or muscle pain can persist up to weeks or months after the acute phase of COVID-19. Since chronic pain is described as a manifestation of real or potential tissue damage and it is identified as a perception influenced by the complex interactions of biological, psychological, and social factors, the issue of COVID-pain should be carefully addressed [112]. Moreover, it cannot be excluded that the disease may exacerbate already present painful manifestations. Furthermore, the triggering of de novo clinical manifestations in survivors must be highly evaluated. For example, it is necessary to consider the new-onset chronic pain in critically ill patients suffering from ARDS [113].

Practical Therapeutic Suggestions
Acute COVID-Pain

- It is treated symptomatically. Acetaminophen or NSAIDs (e.g., ibuprofen for short periods) can be used.
- The use of opioids (unless in ICU patients) should be avoided.
- Vitamin B and neurotropic supplement may be suggested.

2.6 Skeletal Muscle Manifestations

2.6.1 Asthenia and Myalgia

Combined or not with myalgia, asthenia is a frequent symptom in SARS-CoV2 infections. In a systematic review, seven studies reported that myalgia can affect about a quarter of COVID-19 patients [85]. Another analysis found that muscle pain is reported in up to 62% of patients, with a higher percentage in Europe compared to East Asia. It was also indicated that joint pain may affect 10–15% of patients, also as an early symptom of the disease [127]. In a prospective consecutive observational study on 61 consecutive adult patients, of whom 57% admitted to ICU, the most common neurological finding was a motor weakness (34.4%), significantly more prevalent in ICU patients (54%) compared to non-ICU patients (7.7%), $p = 0.002$ [35]. The mechanisms underlying the symptomatology could be linked to an excessive production of proinflammatory cytokines and the hypercatabolic state present during the disease process. In fact, the older age, some comorbidities, such as diabetes and obesity, other symptoms commonly found in these patients, such as anorexia, nausea, and vomiting, induce a muscle wasting that triggers an inflammatory response, and oxidative stress. It can amplify the production of proinflammatory cytokine, leading to a vicious circle, with worsening damage [128].

2.6.2 Skeletal Muscle Injury

Myalgia combined with increased serum creatinine kinase levels is defined as a skeletal muscle injury. This condition was found in most severe cases of COVID-19, especially in presence of higher levels of inflammatory indices and multiorgan failure [128]. A case of rhabdomyolysis with pain, weakness of lower limbs and tenderness on examination, raised levels of serum myoglobin, creatine kinase, lactate dehydrogenase, alanine aminotransferase, and aspartate aminotransferase was also described as a late complication of COVID-19 [129].

In a retrospective analysis on 1099 patients from 552 hospitals in China, myalgia/arthralgia was present in 14.9% of patients and increased creatine kinase levels (≥200 U/L) in 13.7% of patients; the percentage of both clinical and laboratory findings were higher in the most severe patients (17.3% vs. 14.5%, and 19% vs. 12.5%, respectively) [18]. Moreover, a large retrospective study ($n = 351$) showed an increase of CK in 27% of COVID-19 and the levels correlated significantly with inflammation markers and severity of the disease. Nevertheless, compared to a cohort of patients with influenza, only a minority of COVID-19 ICU-admitted patients showed higher CK levels (CK > 1000 U/L) (4.7% vs. 35.7%) [130].

The pathogenesis of the COVID-19-associated skeletal muscle injury needs to be better explained. The acute onset of severe muscle weakness with increased inflammatory markers and very high CK levels may suggest an autoimmune cause of the myopathy, as an expression of a necrotizing autoimmune myositis [131]. On the other hand, direct muscle toxicity of virus cannot be excluded [130].

2.7 Psychiatric Manifestations

As the COVID-19 has been declared a public health emergency, measures to combat the spread of the virus have been adopted by national governments. Some of these measures, such as nation-wide lockdown and social distancing, could represent a psychological burden leading to the occurrence of psychiatric manifestations. Furthermore, the overwhelming flow of information from social media can further worsen the psychosocial impact of pandemic [132–134].

Previous outbreaks have reported many symptoms linked to prolonged quarantine, like irritability, fear of spreading the infection, confusion, anxiety, depression, and obsessive-compulsive behavior, such as repeated temperature checks and sterilization [134]. In this context, the loss of freedom, the separation from the family, the uncertainty about the disease evolution, and the concern for financial losses might induce or worsen in the COVID-19 patients' emotional disturbances, such as depression, anxiety, obsessive behaviors, and insomnia [135, 136].

Notably, the pathophysiological mechanisms of COVID-19 could also be responsible of psychiatric complications. The direct viral effects on CNS, the immune response of the patients with cytokine storm, cerebrovascular injury or, more generally, hypoxic conditions and post-infectious autoimmunity, all could lead to the onset of the clinical picture [132]. Furthermore, the continuous presence of stressful symptoms, such as cough and fever, the side effects of drugs, such as insomnia due to the use of steroids or some psychotic effects of chloroquine, could exacerbate the mental disturbances of more frail patients [58, 62]. Moreover, for patients admitted to hospital, organizational and logistic factors, such as prolonged isolation and separation from the families, personal protective equipment worn by the hospital staff that limits the human contact, the environmental pressure around the patient, and the sleep deprivation might play a central role. On the other hand, concurring psychiatric symptoms can obstacle the respiratory management of COVID-19 patients due to problems of treatment adherence.

Finally, the more severe patients treated in intensive and semi-intensive care units are at higher risk of occurrence of psychiatric symptoms. It is now well known that the management of pain, agitation, and delirium has a positive impact on both in short- and long-term outcomes of ICU patients. Light sedation in most patients can be safely used preventing a long list of problems associated with deeper levels, such as loss of human contact, ICU-acquired weakness, immunosuppression, delirium, and permanent cognitive deficits. Similarly, critical patients can frequently experience pain, either at rest or during routine procedures, with a negative impact on the psychological status during ICU stay and after the discharge. Delirium is a fearful complication and is associated with increased mortality, length of ICU, and hospital stay, as well as development of post-ICU cognitive impairment; its incidence has been reported from 20% to 80% of the critical patients; risk factors are age, dementia, serious illness at admission, history of hypertension, coma and the use of benzodiazepine and opioids [137–140].

It is important to underline that there is a close relationship between agitation, pain, delirium, and their treatment. Moreover, both agitation and pain are risk factor for delirium but also an incorrect treatment could lead to the onset of delirium and the so called Post Intensive Care Syndrome (PICS). On this topic, international guidelines recommended a structured approach. Each approach focus based on the following points [137–139, 141]:

1. A prevention strategy aimed to recognize and remove all the possible risk factors.
2. The use of monitoring tools to evaluate the proper management of pain, agitation, and delirium and to identify early the occurrence of such complications.
3. The use of the more appropriate pharmacologic interventions and, whenever possible, the non-pharmacologic approaches. In this regard light sedation using short acting sedatives, a multimodal opioid sparing analgesia, a careful assessment for delirium using validated tools and its treatment with non-pharmacologic, and pharmacologic approaches are valid options to be introduced in the clinical practice.

A study on medical records from a US network of health care organizations on 9086 patients with neuropsychiatric manifestations, of whom 73.7% outpatients and 26.3% inpatients, demonstrated a variety of manifestations: anxiety and related disorders (4.6%), mood disorders (3.8%), sleep disorders (3.4%), emotional state symptoms and signs (0.8%), and suicidal ideation (0.2%) [58]. In another study on 707 hospitalized non-ICU patients older >50 years, the incidence of delirium was 33%, of whom 12% were delirious on admission. In these patients, delirium was associated with in-hospital death with an adjusted Odds Ratio [aOR] of 1.75 (95% CI = 1.15–2.66) and with increased length of stay, admission to intensive care, and ventilator utilization [142]. Another report from Italy on 852 non-ICU patients showed an incidence of delirium of 11%; in this study, delirium was positively associated with age and use of antipsychotic drugs with higher mortality (57% vs. 30%) [143].

Some atypical presentations have been described in the literature. In a case report a 70-years-old man, without a story of cognitive deficit, at hospital admission revealed cognitive and perception problems, with disturbances in memory and orientation but without any other complaints; brain; TC excluded brain pathology, while a PCR test for SARS-CoV-2 was positive; a typical symptomatology appeared after 5 days of hospitalization; hydroxychloroquine, favipiravir, tocilizumab, prednisolone, and enoxaparin were started with a dramatic improvement of clinical and laboratory parameters [144]. In another case, a 94-year-old man with schizoaffective disorders was admitted to hospital drowsy, disorientated, trying to undress himself and resisting care and signs of respiratory infection; he was treated with antibiotics and fluids; after 3 days his clinical and CT findings worsened and he died after 5 days; a postmortem nasopharyngeal swab was positive for SARS-CoV-2 RNA [145].

Some studies confirmed the higher prevalence of delirium in ICU patients with COVID-19 compared to COVID-19 non-ICU inpatients [142, 143]. These findings were confirmed by a study on 150 ICU patients with COVID-19 that showed a prevalence of delirium of 79.5%, of whom 86.6% with a hyperactive form; the duration of ventilation was significantly longer in patients with delirium, while the mortality higher but did not reach statistical significance [146].

Patients with psychiatric complications could have a higher incidence of psychiatric symptoms at the discharge. An observational series on 58 patients showed that agitation was present in 69% and confusion in 65% of patients on admission in ICU, or at the suspension of sedation and neuromuscular blockade. In this series, a third of the discharged subjects showed a dysexecutive syndrome (inattention, disorientation, or poorly organized movements in response to command) [44].

In ICU patients, the measures to prevent delirium and improve the psychophysical outcome at discharge (ICU liberation and similar initiatives) are presented in the mnemonic form, such as ABCDEF bundle (A: assess, prevent, and manage pain; B: both spontaneous awakening trials and spontaneous breathing trials; C: choice of analgesia and sedation; D: delirium: assess, prevent, and manage; E: early mobility and exercise; F: family engagement and empowerment) [147] or eCASH concept (early Comfort using Analgesia, minimal Sedation, and maximal Human care) [138]. Most of the abovementioned measures could be challenging in COVID-19 patients, mainly when in ICU. Nevertheless, some interventions could aid to prevent delirium and improve the long-term physical and psychological conditions of these patients [141].

The shortage of clinician resources could reduce the interest for some of the abovementioned measures, such as early mobility, to spend more time for others, such as pain and sedation management. Furthermore, the shortage of some sedatives during pandemic could explain the increased use of benzodiazepines, while the presence of less trained staff could lead to a choice of deep levels of sedation and neuromuscular block for a prolonged time. The use of some items of validated scales, such as facial expression or body movements, could aid to adjust the level of analgesia. Furthermore, maintaining a systematic detection of pain could allow to point out the development of peripheral neuropathies from viral invasion. The use of a protocolized approach to daily target of sedation using validated scales and titrating the dose to the ventilator-patient synchrony and the use, whenever possible, of depth sedation monitoring devices could prevent the unnecessary prolonged deep sedations. Furthermore, the heavy workload and the limitation to the access of physiotherapists could generate the ICU-acquired weakness and compromise physical functions at the discharge; passive physiotherapy and virtual consultation to guide physiotherapy and rehabilitation could be considered to limit such complications [148].

The usual practice of open-ICU, allowing the parents to enter and involve them in the care of the patients and prevention of delirium has been restricted because of the needing for extreme isolation. Nevertheless, delirium is associated with higher incidence adverse events, such as self-extubation, and to a worse outcome at the discharge, so every effort should be made to prevent, recognize, and adequately treat this complication. It is suggested for wakeful patients the daily use of telephone or video call with the family and friends and family photos [148]. Other factors, such as the elevated environmental noise during the day and night with disruption of sleep-wake cycle, the systematic use of personal protective equipment and contact distancing, the occurrence of complications, such as cerebrovascular disease and sepsis, could further increase the incidence of delirium in COVID-19 patients. It is crucial to provide a regular screening of delirium using validated scale, such as CAM-ICU, and the non-pharmacological interventions, such as glasses and hearing aids, reorientation measure, and reduction of nocturnal light and noise [141, 148].

The need of social distancing and the increase of workload has been reduced the interprofessional confrontation; alternative mode of interactions, such as virtual participation, could overcome this kind of problem. The use of less trained staff, due to an increased number of ICU beds in the hospital, could lead to a suboptimal care and a reduced use of bundles; it seems possible to resolve this point by adopting a model of on-field training, guidance, and coaching managed by experienced clinicians [141, 148].

A multi-center international cohort study including 2088 COVID-19 ICU patients across 14 countries confirms most of the abovementioned observations. 84% of participant hospitals added a mean of 24 (12–39) additional ICU beds; 99% of sites had restricted visitation due to pandemic, but 96% had a facilitated virtual contact between the patients and the family or friends; all the sites had a level of sedation assessment tool (mainly Richmond Agitation-Sedation Scale) and 90% had a protocol to identify delirium (mainly CAM-ICU) but only 68% a protocol for its management. In 42% of participant hospitals there was a shortage of available resource (79% critical care providers, 72% personal protective equipment, 55% ventilators, 38% sedatives); ARDS diagnosis was made in 97.9% of patients, invasive mechanical ventilation was used in 66.9% and non-invasive ventilation in 8.3% of patients; opioids infusion was used in 79.5% benzodiazepine in 74% (for a median of 7 days), propofol in 70.9%, dexmedetomidine in 44.1%, and clonidine in 9.1% of patients. The prevalence of coma was 81.6% (mean duration of 10 days) and the prevalence of delirium was 54.9% (mean duration 3 days) of the patients [149]. The authors evaluated the degree of implementation of ABCDEF bundle: pain was assessed at least once in 73% of eligible days; the evaluation of spontaneous awakening trial and spontaneous breathing trial was, respectively, done in the 23.8% and 22.8%, respectively; delirium was evaluated in 82.9% of eligible days; sedation-agitation was evaluated in 98.1% of eligible days but avoidance of benzodiazepine was adopted only in 52.4% of eligible days; some type of early mobility was performed only in 33.9% and family engagement in 17% of eligible days. The authors concluded that clinicians should adhere to evidence-based guidelines for the COVID-19 patients in similar manner to those without disease, mainly in the choice of an adequate sedation regime [149].

An Italian multidisciplinary group has underlined the importance of permitting visits in ICUs even during the COVID-19 pandemic. Some benefits can be summarized in a reduction of stress and depression for the patients and families, the increased compliance to care and prevention of delirium, and help in decision making and reduction of moral distress for healthcare teams. In this paper the authors suggest some tips, indicating the necessary rules for an effective and safe ICU opening [150].

Practical Therapeutic Suggestions

According to guidelines, it must be performed [141]:

- A careful pain management
- A protocol to identify pain, agitation, and delirium
- A protocol to prevent delirium, by:
  - Non-pharmacological strategies. For example, protocol for sedation, glasses and hearing aids, reorientation measure, and reduction of nocturnal light and noise.
  - Pharmacological approaches. Dexmedetomidine: although not recommended, low doses (e.g., 0.1 μg/kg per hour) may reduce ICU-delirium occurrence
- A protocol to treat delirium, by:
  - Haloperidol (2–10 mg IV every 6 h), but recommended for not routinely using (especially in hyperactive form)
  - Olanzapine (IM 5–10 mg; max: 30 mg/d), risperidone (0.5–8 mg), quetiapine (orally 50 mg; max 400 mg/d), and ziprasidone (IM 10 mg; max: 40 mg/d)
  - Dexmedetomidine: in adults under mechanical ventilation, especially when hyperactive manifestations preclude weaning
- A family/caregiver/friend-centered "visitation" policy.

2.8 Conclusions

Acute neurological manifestations of COVID-19 involving the CNS or the PNS configure a chapter of paramount importance. Obviously, many gaps need to be filled to fully understand the pathogenetic mechanisms, the risk factors, the long-term consequences of the multiple clinical expressions of neuro-COVID. Despite the amount of research produced on the subject, further preclinical studies, and clinical research with the contribution of epidemiological data, is necessary. In the meantime, thanks to prospective and retrospective observational studies, but also case reports and case series (useful for rare complications and those with anomalous presentation), a picture of the phenomenon is beginning to be drawn. Evidence-based medicine studies require "high quality" data, and this aim is often achievable through multi-center research. In this regard, COVID-19 represents an incredible opportunity to establish lasting scientific collaborations, with alliances between various biomedical and no-biomedical figures such as bioinformatics, statisticians, and experts in artificial intelligence who belong to the most disparate fields of research.

References

1. Wu Z, McGoogan JM. Characteristics of and important lessons from the coronavirus disease 2019 (COVID-19) outbreak in China: summary of a report of 72 314 cases from the Chinese Center for Disease Control and Prevention. JAMA. 2020;323(13):1239–42. https://doi.org/10.1001/jama.2020.2648.
2. Epidemiology Working Group for NCIP Epidemic Response, Chinese Center for Disease Control and Prevention. The epidemiological characteristics of an outbreak of 2019 novel coronavirus diseases (COVID-19) in China. Zhonghua Liu Xing Bing Xue Za Zhi. 2020;41(2):145–51. https://doi.org/10.3760/cma.j.issn.0254-6450.2020.02.003.
3. Docherty AB, Harrison EM, Green CA, et al. Features of 20 133 UK patients in hospital with covid-19 using the ISARIC WHO clinical characterisation protocol: prospective observational cohort study. BMJ. 2020;369:m1985. https://doi.org/10.1136/bmj.m1985.
4. Lechien JR, Chiesa-Estomba CM, et al. Clinical and epidemiological characteristics of 1420 European patients with mild-to-moderate coronavirus disease 2019. J Intern Med. 2020;288(3):335–44. https://doi.org/10.1111/joim.13089.
5. Rodriguez-Morales AJ, Cardona-Ospina JA, Gutiérrez-Ocampo E, et al. Clinical, laboratory and imaging features of COVID-19: a systematic review and meta-analysis. Travel Med Infect Dis. 2020;34:101623. https://doi.org/10.1016/j.tmaid.2020.101623.
6. Yang J, Zhenga Y, Gou X, et al. Prevalence of comorbidities and its effects in patients infected with SARS-CoV-2: a systematic review and meta-analysis. Int J Infect Diseases. 2020;94:91–5.
7. Davoodi L, Jafarpour H, Taghavi M, et al. COVID-19 presented with deep vein thrombosis: an unusual presenting. J Investig Med High Impact Case Rep. 2020;8:2324709620931239. https://doi.org/10.1177/2324709620931239.
8. Klopfenstein T, Kadiane-Oussou NJ, Royer PY, et al. Diarrhea: an underestimated symptom in coronavirus disease 2019. Clin Res Hepatol Gastroenterol. 2020;44(3):282–3. https://doi.org/10.1016/j.clinre.2020.04.002.
9. Velev V, Popov M, Velikov P, et al. COVID-19 and gastrointestinal injury: a brief systematic review and data from Bulgaria. Infez Med. 2020;28(Suppl. 1):37–41.

10. Aloysius MM, Thatti A, Gupta A, et al. COVID-19 presenting as acute pancreatitis. Pancreatology. 2020;20(5):1026–7. https://doi.org/10.1016/j.pan.2020.05.003.
11. Wander P, Epstein M, Bernstein D. COVID-19 presenting as acute hepatitis. Am J Gastroenterol. 2020;115(6):941–2. https://doi.org/10.14309/ajg.0000000000000660.
12. Sachdeva M, Gianotti R. Cutaneous manifestations of COVID-19: report of three cases and a review of literature. J Dermatol Sci. 2020;98:75–81.
13. Struyf T, Deeks JJ, Dinnes J, et al. Signs and symptoms to determine if a patient presenting in primary care or hospital outpatient settings has COVID-19 disease. Cochrane Database Syst Rev. 2020;7:CD013665. https://doi.org/10.1002/14651858.CD013665.
14. Wiersinga WJ, Rhodes A, Cheng AC, et al. Pathophysiology, transmission, diagnosis, and treatment of coronavirus disease 2019 (COVID-19). A Review. JAMA. 2020;324(8):782–93.
15. Krishnan A, Hamilton JP, Alqahtani SA, et al. A narrative review of coronavirus disease 2019 (COVID-19): clinical, epidemiological characteristics, and systemic manifestations. Intern Emerg Med. 2021;16:1–16. https://doi.org/10.1007/s11739-020-02616-5.
16. Cummings MG, Baldwin MR, Abrams D, et al. Epidemiology, clinical course, and outcomes of critically ill adults with COVID-19 in new York City: a prospective cohort study. Lancet. 2020;395:1763–70.
17. Grasselli G, Greco M, Zanella A, et al. Risk factors associated with mortality among patients with COVID-19 in intensive care units in Lombardy, Italy. JAMA Intern Med. 2020;180(10):1345–55.
18. Guan WJ, Ni ZY, Hu Y, et al. Clinical characteristics of coronavirus disease 2019 in China. N Engl J Med. 2020;382:1708–20.
19. Johns Hopkins Coronavirus Resource Center. Mortality analyses. updated on Thursday, January 21, 2021 at 03:00 AM EST. https://coronavirus.jhu.edu/data/mortality
20. Onder G, Rezza G, Brusaferro S. Case-fatality rate and characteristics of patients dying in relation to COVID-19 in Italy. JAMA. 2020;323(18):1775–6.
21. Lau KK, Yu WC, Chu CM, et al. Possible central nervous system infection by SARS coronavirus. Emerg Infect Dis. 2004;10(2):342–4. https://doi.org/10.3201/eid1002.030638.
22. Ng Kee Kwong KC, Mehta PR, et al. COVID-19, SARS and MERS: a neurological perspective. J Clin Neurosci. 2020;77:13–6. https://doi.org/10.1016/j.jocn.2020.04.124.
23. Nilsson A, Edner N, Albert J, Ternhag A. Fatal encephalitis associated with coronavirus OC43 in an immunocompromised child. Infect Dis (Auckl). 2020;52:419–22.
24. Mao L, Jin H, Wang M, et al. Neurologic manifestations of hospitalized patients with coronavirus disease 2019 in Wuhan, China. JAMA Neurol. 2020;77(6):683–90. https://doi.org/10.1001/jamaneurol.2020.1127.
25. Chou SHY, Beghi E, Helbok R, et al. Global incidence of neurological manifestations among patients hospitalized with COVID-19—a report for the GCS-NeuroCOVID consortium and the ENERGY consortium. JAMA Netw Open. 2021;4(5):e2112131. https://doi.org/10.1001/jamanetworkopen.2021.12131.
26. Zubair AS, McAlpine LS, et al. Neuropathogenesis and neurologic manifestations of the coronaviruses in the age of coronavirus disease 2019 a review. JAMA Neurol. 2020;77(8):1018–27.
27. Förster M, Weyers V, Küry P, et al. Neurological manifestations of severe acute respiratory syndrome coronavirus 2-a controversy 'gone viral'. Brain Commun. 2020;2(2):fcaa149. https://doi.org/10.1093/braincomms/fcaa149.
28. Ahmad I, Rathore FA. Neurological manifestations and complications of COVID-19: a literature review. J Clin Neurosci. 2020;77:8–12. https://doi.org/10.1016/j.jocn.2020.05.017.
29. Ratajczak J, Wysoczynski M, Hayek F, et al. Membrane-derived microvesicles: important and underappreciated mediators of cell-to-cell communication. Leukemia. 2006;20:1487–95.
30. Özdag Acarli AN, Samanci B, et al. (2020) coronavirus disease 2019 (COVID-19) from the point of view of neurologists: observation of neurological findings and symptoms during the combat against a pandemic. Arch Neuropsychiatry. 2020;57:154–9.
31. Matschke J, Lütgehetmann M, Hagel C, et al. Neuropathology of patients with COVID-19 in Germany: a post-mortem case series. Lancet Neurol. 2020;19(11):919–29. https://doi.org/10.1016/S1474-4422(20)30308-2.

32. Solomon IH, Normandin E, et al. Neuropathological features of Covid-19. N Engl J Med. 2020;383:10.
33. Reichard RR, Kashani KB, Boire NA, et al. Neuropathology of COVID-19: a spectrum of vascular and acute disseminated encephalomyelitis (ADEM)-like pathology. Acta Neuropathol. 2020;140(1):1–6. https://doi.org/10.1007/s00401-020-02166-2.
34. Yu H, Sun T, Feng J. Complications and pathophysiology of COVID-19 in the nervous system. Front Neurol. 2020;11:573421. https://doi.org/10.3389/fneur.2020.573421.
35. Nersesjan V, Amiri M, Lebech AM, et al. Central and peripheral nervous system complications of COVID-19: a prospective tertiary center cohort with 3-month follow-up. J Neurol. 2021:1–19. https://doi.org/10.1007/s00415-020-10380-x.
36. Berlit P, Bösel J, Gahn G, et al. Neurological manifestations of COVID-19 - guideline of the German society of neurology. Neurol Res Pract. 2020;2:51. https://doi.org/10.1186/s42466-020-00097-7.
37. Meppiel E, Peiffer-Smadja N, Maury A, et al. Neurologic manifestations associated with COVID-19: a multicentre registry. Clin Microbiol Infect. S1198-743X(20)30698-4. 2020; https://doi.org/10.1016/j.cmi.2020.11.005.
38. Kacem I, Gharbi A, Harizi C, et al. Characteristics, onset, and evolution of neurological symptoms in patients with COVID-19. Neurol Sci. 2021;42(1):39–46. https://doi.org/10.1007/s10072-020-04866-9.
39. Borges do Nascimento IJ, Cacic N, Abdulazeem HM, et al. Novel coronavirus infection (COVID-19) in humans: a scoping review and meta-analysis. J Clin Med. 2020;9(4):941. https://doi.org/10.3390/jcm9040941.
40. Islam MA, Alam SS, Kundu S, et al C (2020) Prevalence of headache in patients with coronavirus disease 2019 (COVID-19): a systematic review and meta-analysis of 14,275 patients. Front Neurol 11:562634. https://doi.org/10.3389/fneur.2020.562634
41. Pinzon RT, Wijaya VO, Buana RB, et al. Neurologic characteristics in coronavirus disease 2019 (COVID-19): a systematic review and meta-analysis. Front Neurol. 2020;11:565. https://doi.org/10.3389/fneur.2020.00565.
42. Uygun Ö, Ertaş M, Ekizoğlu E, et al. J Headache Pain. 2020;21:121. https://doi.org/10.1186/s10194-020-01188-1.
43. Viola P, Ralli M, Pisani D, et al. Tinnitus and equilibrium disorders in COVID-19 patients: preliminary results. Eur Arch Otorhinolaryngol. 2020;23:1–6. https://doi.org/10.1007/s00405-020-06440-7.
44. Helms J, Kremer S, Merdji H, et al. Neurologic features in severe SARS-CoV-2 infection. N Engl J Med. 2020;382(23):2268–70. https://doi.org/10.1056/NEJMc2008597.
45. Slooter AJC, Otte WM, Devlin JW, et al. Updated nomenclature of delirium and acute encephalopathy: statement of 10 societies. Intensive Care Med. 2020;46:1020–2.
46. Cascella M, Fiore M, Leone S, et al. Current controversies and future perspectives on treatment of intensive care unit delirium in adults. World J Crit Care Med. 2019;8(3):18–27. https://doi.org/10.5492/wjccm.v8.i3.18.
47. Cascella M, Bimonte S. The role of general anesthetics and the mechanisms of hippocampal and extra-hippocampal dysfunctions in the genesis of postoperative cognitive dysfunction. Neural Regen Res. 2017;12(11):1780–5. https://doi.org/10.4103/1673-5374.219032.
48. Cascella M, Muzio MR, Bimonte S, et al. Postoperative delirium and postoperative cognitive dysfunction: updates in pathophysiology, potential translational approaches to clinical practice and further research perspectives. Minerva Anestesiol. 2018;84(2):246–60. https://doi.org/10.23736/S0375-9393.17.12146-2.
49. Krishnan V, Leung LY, Caplan LR. A neurologist's approach to delirium: diagnosis and management of toxic metabolic encephalopathies. Eur J Intern Med. 2014;25(2):112–6. https://doi.org/10.1016/j.ejim.2013.11.010.
50. Garg RK, Paliwal VK, Gupta A. Encephalopathy in patients with COVID-19: a review. J Med Virol. 2021;93(1):206–22. https://doi.org/10.1002/jmv.26207.
51. Gewirtz AN, Gao V, Parauda SC. Posterior reversible encephalopathy syndrome. Curr Pain Headache Rep. 2021;25:19. https://doi.org/10.1007/s11916-020-00932-1.

52. Kishfy L, Casasola M, Banankhah P, et al. Posterior reversible encephalopathy syndrome (PRES) as a neurological association in severe Covid19. J Neurol Sci. 2020;414:116943.
53. Parauda SC, Gao V, Gewirtz AN, et al. Posterior reversible encephalopathy syndrome in patients with COVID-19. J Neurol Sci. 2020;416:117019. https://doi.org/10.1016/j.jns.2020.117019.
54. Anzalone N, Castellano A, Scotti R, et al. Multifocal laminar cortical brain lesions: a consistent MRI finding in neuro-COVID-19 patients. J Neurol. 2020;267(10):2806–9. https://doi.org/10.1007/s00415-020-09966-2.
55. Colombo A, Martinelli Boneschi F, Beretta S, et al. Posterior reversible encephalopathy syndrome and COVID-19: a series of 6 cases from Lombardy, Italy. eNeurologicalSci. 2021;22:100306. https://doi.org/10.1016/j.ensci.2020.100306.
56. Franceschi AM, Ahmed O, Giliberto L, et al. Hemorrhagic posterior reversible encephalopathy syndrome as a manifestation of COVID-19 infection. AJNR Am J Neuroradiol. 2020;41(7):1173–6. https://doi.org/10.3174/ajnr.A6595.
57. Dias DA, de Brito LA, Neves LO, et al. Hemorrhagic PRES: an unusual neurologic manifestation in two COVID-19 patients. Arq Neuropsiquiatr. 2020;78(11):739–40. https://doi.org/10.1590/0004-282X20200184.
58. Nalleballe K, Reddy Onteddu S, et al. Spectrum of neuropsychiatric manifestations in COVID-19. Brain Behav Immun. 2020;88:71–4. https://doi.org/10.1016/j.bbi.2020.06.020.
59. Khedr EM, Shoybb A, Mohammaden M, et al. Acute symptomatic seizures and COVID-19: hospital-based study. Epilepsy Res. 2021;174:106650. https://doi.org/10.1016/j.eplepsyres.2021.106650.
60. Asadi-Pooya AA, Simani L, Shahisavandi M, et al. COVID-19, de novo seizures, and epilepsy: a systematic review. Neurol Sci. 2021;42(2):415–31. https://doi.org/10.1007/s10072-020-04932-2.
61. Nikbakht F, Mohammadkhanizadeh A, Mohammadi E. How does the COVID-19 cause seizure and epilepsy in patients? The potential mechanisms. Mult Scler Relat Disord. 2020;46:102535. https://doi.org/10.1016/j.msard.2020.102535.
62. Acar T, Demirel EA, Afsar N, et al. The COVID-19 from neurological overview. Turk J Neurol. 2020;26:58–108. https://doi.org/10.4274/tnd.2020.73669.
63. Cabezudo-García P, Ciano-Petersen NL, Mena-Vázquez N, et al. Incidence and case fatality rate of COVID-19 in patients with active epilepsy. Neurology. 2020;95(10):e1417–25. https://doi.org/10.1212/WNL.0000000000010033.
64. Kuroda N. Epilepsy and COVID-19: associations and important considerations. Epilepsy Behav. 2020;108:107122.
65. Nannoni S, de Groot R, Bell S, et al. Stroke in COVID-19: a systematic review and meta-analysis. Int J Stroke. 2021;16(2):137–49. https://doi.org/10.1177/1747493020972922.
66. Ghosh R, Roy D, Mandal A, et al. Cerebral venous thrombosis in COVID-19. Diabetes Metab Syndr. 2021;15(3):1039–45. https://doi.org/10.1016/j.dsx.2021.04.026.
67. Bridwell R, Long B, Gottlieb M. Neurologic complications of COVID-19. Am J Emerg Med. 2020;38(7):1549.e3–7. https://doi.org/10.1016/j.ajem.2020.05.024.
68. Wu X, Wu W, Pan W, et al. Acute necrotizing encephalopathy: an underrecognized clinicoradiologic disorder. Mediators Inflamm. 2015:792578. https://doi.org/10.1155/2015/792578.
69. Poyiadji N, Shahin G, Noujaim D, et al. COVID-19-associated acute hemorrhagic necrotizing encephalopathy: imaging features. Radiology. 2020;296(2):E119–20. https://doi.org/10.1148/radiol.2020201187.
70. Virhammar J, Kumlien E, Fällmar D, et al. Acute necrotizing encephalopathy with SARS-CoV-2 RNA confirmed in cerebrospinal fluid. Neurology. 2020;95(10):445–9. https://doi.org/10.1212/WNL.0000000000010250.
71. Haroon KH, Patro SN, Hussain S, et al. Multiple microbleeds: a serious neurological manifestation in a critically ill COVID-19 patient. Case Rep Neurol. 2020;12(3):373–7. https://doi.org/10.1159/000512322.
72. Parsons T, Banks S, Bae C, et al. COVID-19-associated acute disseminated encephalomyelitis (ADEM). J Neurol. 2020;267(10):2799–802. https://doi.org/10.1007/s00415-020-09951-9.

73. Handa R, Nanda S, Prasad A, et al. Covid-19-associated acute haemorrhagic leukoencephalomyelitis. Neurol Sci. 2020;41(11):3023–6. https://doi.org/10.1007/s10072-020-04703-z.
74. Varadan B, Shankar A, Rajakumar A, et al. Acute hemorrhagic leukoencephalitis in a COVID-19 patient—a case report with literature review. Neuroradiology. 2021:1–9. https://doi.org/10.1007/s00234-021-02667-1.
75. Ladopoulos T, Zand R, Shahjouei S, et al. COVID-19: neuroimaging features of a pandemic. J Neuroimaging. 2021:1–16. https://doi.org/10.1111/jon.12819.
76. Zhao K, Huang J, Dai D, et al. Acute myelitis after SARS-CoV-2 infection: a case report. medRxiv. 2020.03.16.20035105. 2020; https://doi.org/10.1101/2020.03.16.20035105.
77. AlKetbi R, AlNuaimi D, AlMulla M, et al. Acute myelitis as a neurological complication of Covid-19: a case report and MRI findings. Radiol Case Rep. 2020;15(9):1591–5.
78. Munz M, Wessendorf S, Koretsis G, et al. Acute transverse myelitis after COVID-19 pneumonia. J Neurol. 2020;26:1–2.
79. Rodríguez de Antonio LA, Gonzalez-Suarez I, Fernandez-Barriuso I, et al. Para-infectious anti-GD2/GD3 IgM myelitis during the Covid-19 pandemic: case report and literature review. Mult Scler Relat Disord. 2021;49:102783. https://doi.org/10.1016/j.msard.2021.102783.
80. Cirulli ET, Barrett KMS, Riffle S, et al. Long-term COVID-19 symptoms in a large unselected population. medRxiv. 2020; https://doi.org/10.1101/2020.10.07.20208702.
81. Tuma R, Guedes BF, Carra R, et al. Clinical, cerebrospinal fluid, and neuroimaging findings in COVID-19 encephalopathy: a case series. Neurol Sci. 2021;42(2):479–89. https://doi.org/10.1007/s10072-020-04946-w.
82. Vogrig A, Gigli GL, Bnà C, Morassi M. Stroke in patients with COVID-19: clinical and neuroimaging characteristics. Neurosci Lett. 2021;743:135564. https://doi.org/10.1016/j.neulet.2020.135564.
83. Alshebri MS, Alshouimi RA, Alhumidi HA, et al. Neurological complications of SARS-CoV, MERS-CoV, and COVID-19. SN Compr Clin Med. 2020;16:1–11. https://doi.org/10.1007/s42399-020-00589-2.
84. Tan YK, Goh C, Leow AST, et al. COVID-19 and ischemic stroke: a systematic review and meta-summary of the literature. J Thromb Thrombol. 2020;50(3):587–95. https://doi.org/10.1007/s11239-020-02228-y.
85. Nepal G, Rehrig JH, et al. Neurological manifestations of COVID-19. a systematic review. Crit Care. 2020;24:421. https://doi.org/10.1186/s13054-020-03121-z.
86. Fraiman P, Godeiro Junior C, Moro E, et al. COVID-19 and cerebrovascular diseases: a systematic review and perspectives for stroke management. Front Neurol. 2020;11:574694. https://doi.org/10.3389/fneur.2020.574694.
87. Hernandez-Fernandez F, Sandoval Valencia H, et al. Cerebrovascular disease in patients with COVID-19: neuroimaging, histological and clinical description. Brain. 2020;143(10):3089–103. https://doi.org/10.1093/brain/awaa239.
88. Mendes A, Herrmann FR, Genton L, et al. Incidence, characteristics and clinical relevance of acute stroke in old patients hospitalized with COVID-19. BMC Geriatr. 2021;21(1):52. https://doi.org/10.1186/s12877-021-02006-2.
89. Collantes MEV, Espiritu AI, Sy MCC, Anlacan VMM, Jamora RDG. Neurological manifestations in COVID-19 infection: a systematic review and meta-analysis. Can J Neurol Sci. 2021;48(1):66–76. https://doi.org/10.1017/cjn.2020.146.
90. Yaghi S, Ishida K, Torres J, et al. SARS-CoV-2 and stroke in a New York healthcare system. Stroke. 2020;51(7):2002–11. https://doi.org/10.1161/STROKEAHA.120.030335.
91. Baldini T, Asioli GM, Romoli M, et al. Cerebral venous thrombosis and severe acute respiratory syndrome coronavirus-2 infection: a systematic review and meta-analysis. Eur J Neurol. 2021; https://doi.org/10.1111/ene.14727.
92. Wang Z, Yang Y, Liang X, et al. COVID-19 associated ischemic stroke and hemorrhagic stroke: incidence, potential pathological mechanism, and management. Front Neurol. 2020;11:571996. https://doi.org/10.3389/fneur.2020.571996.
93. Koralnik IJ, Tyler KL. COVID-19: a global threat to the nervous system. Ann Neurol. 2020;88:1–11.

94. Robles L. Bilateral large vessel occlusion causing massive ischemic stroke in a COVID-19 patient. J Stroke Cerebrovasc Dis. 2021;30(3):105609.
95. Dhamoon MS, Thaler A, Gururangan K, et al. Acute cerebrovascular events with COVID-19 infection. Stroke. 2021;52:48–56.
96. Morassi M, Bigni B, Cobelli M, et al. Bilateral carotid artery dissection in a SARS-CoV-2 infected patient: causality or coincidence? J Neurol. 2020;267(10):2812–4. https://doi.org/10.1007/s00415-020-09984-0.
97. Sharifian-Dorche M, Huot P, Osherov M, et al. Neurological complications of coronavirus infection; a comparative review and lessons learned during the COVID-19 pandemic. J Neurol Sci. 2020;417:117085. https://doi.org/10.1016/j.jns.2020.117085.
98. Katz JM, Libman RB, Wang JJ, et al. Cerebrovascular complications of COVID-19. Stroke. 2020;51(9):e227–31. https://doi.org/10.1161/STROKEAHA.120.031265.
99. Ntaios G, Michel P, Georgiopoulos G, et al. Characteristics and outcomes in patients with COVID-19 and acute ischemic stroke. The global COVID-19 stroke registry. Stroke. 2020;51:e254–8. https://doi.org/10.1161/STROKEAHA.120.031208.
100. Morassi M, Bagatto D, Cobelli M, et al. Stroke in patients with SARS-CoV-2 infection: case series. J Neurol. 2020;267(8):2185–92. https://doi.org/10.1007/s00415-020-09885-2.
101. Fuentes B, de Leciñana MA, García-Madrona S, et al. Stroke acute management and outcomes during the COVID-19 outbreak. A Cohort Study from the Madrid Stroke Network. Stroke. 2021;52:552–62. https://doi.org/10.1161/STROKEAHA.120.031769.
102. Zhao J, Li H, Kung D, et al. Impact of the COVID-19 epidemic on stroke care and potential solutions. Stroke. 2020;51(7):1996–2001. https://doi.org/10.1161/STROKEAHA.120.030225.
103. Moriguchi T, Harii N, Goto J, et al. A first case of meningitis/encephalitis associated with SARS-Coronavirus-2. Int J Infect Dis. 2020;94:55–8. https://doi.org/10.1016/j.ijid.2020.03.062.
104. Grimaldi S, Lagarde S, Harlé JR, et al. Autoimmune encephalitis concomitant with SARS-CoV-2 infection: insight from 18F-FDG PET imaging and neuronal autoantibodies. J Nucl Med. 2020;61(12):1726–9. https://doi.org/10.2967/jnumed.120.249292.
105. Huo L, Xu KL, Wang H. Clinical features of SARS-CoV-2-associated encephalitis and meningitis amid COVID-19 pandemic. World J Clin Cases. 2021;9(5):1058–78. https://doi.org/10.12998/wjcc.v9.i5.1058.
106. Zhang T, Rodricks MB, Hirsh E. COVID-19-associated acute disseminated encephalomyelitis: a case report. medRxiv. 2020.04.16.20068148. 2020; https://doi.org/10.1101/2020.04.16.20068148.
107. Mutiawati E, Fahriani M, Mamada SS, et al. Anosmia and dysgeusia in SARS-CoV-2 infection: incidence and effects on COVID-19 severity and mortality, and the possible pathobiology mechanisms—a systematic review and metaanalysis. F1000Res. 2021;10:40. https://doi.org/10.12688/f1000research.28393.1.
108. Finsterer L, Scorza FA. Guillain-Barre syndrome in 220 patients with COVID-19. Egypt J Neurol Psychiatry Neurosurg. 2021;57:55. https://doi.org/10.1186/s41983-021-00310-7.
109. Jiang F, Yang WL, Wang JW, et al. Pain during and after coronavirus disease 2019: Chinese perspectives. Pain Rep. 2021;6(1):e931. https://doi.org/10.1097/PR9.0000000000000931.
110. Rowbotham MC, Arendt-Nielsen L. A year like no other: introduction to a special issue on COVID-19 and pain. Pain Rep. 2021;6(1):e915. https://doi.org/10.1097/PR9.0000000000000915.
111. Attal N, Martinez V, Bouhassira D. The potential for increased prevalence of neuropathic pain after the Covid 19 pandemic. Pain Rep. 2021;6:e884. https://doi.org/10.1097/PR9.0000000000000884.
112. Cuomo A, Bimonte S, Forte CA, Botti G, Cascella M. Multimodal approaches and tailored therapies for pain management: the trolley analgesic model. J Pain Res. 2019;12:711–4. https://doi.org/10.2147/JPR.S178910.
113. Vittori A, Lerman J, Cascella M, et al. COVID-19 pandemic acute respiratory distress syndrome survivors: pain after the storm? Anesth Analg. 2020;131(1):117–9. https://doi.org/10.1213/ANE.0000000000004914.

114. Lima MA, Silva MTT, Soares CN, et al. Peripheral facial nerve palsy associated with COVID-19. J Neurovirol. 2020;26(6):941–4. https://doi.org/10.1007/s13365-020-00912-6.
115. Meng X, Deng Y, Dai Z, et al. COVID-19 and anosmia: a review based on up-to-date knowledge. Am J Otolaryngol. 2020;41(5):102581. https://doi.org/10.1016/j.amjoto.2020.102581.
116. Rahman A, Niloofa R, De Zoysa IM, et al. Neurological manifestations in COVID-19: a narrative review. SAGE Open Med. 2020;8:2050312120957925. https://doi.org/10.1177/2050312120957925.
117. Lechien JR, Chiesa-Estomba CM, Beckers E, et al. Prevalence and 6-month recovery of olfactory dysfunction: a multicentre study of 1363 COVID-19 patients. J Intern Med doi. 2021; https://doi.org/10.1111/joim.13209.
118. Lechien JR, Chiesa-Estomba CM, De Siati DR, et al. Olfactory and gustatory dysfunctions as a clinical presentation of mild-to-moderate forms of the coronavirus disease (COVID-19): a multicenter European study. Eur Arch Otorhinolaryngol. 2020;277(8):2251–61. https://doi.org/10.1007/s00405-020-05965-1.
119. Sriwastava S, Kataria S, Tandon M, et al. Guillain Barré syndrome and its variants as a manifestation of COVID-19: a systematic review of case reports and case series. J Neurol Sci. 2021;420:117263. https://doi.org/10.1016/j.jns.2020.117263.
120. Abu-Rumeileh S, Abdelhak A, Foschi M, et al. Guillain-Barré syndrome spectrum associated with COVID-19: an up-to-date systematic review of 73 cases. J Neurol. 2020:1–38. https://doi.org/10.1007/s00415-020-10124-x.
121. Zhao H, Shen D, Zhou H, et al. Guillain-Barré syndrome associated with SARS-CoV-2 infection: causality or coincidence? Lancet Neurol. 2020;19(5):383–4. https://doi.org/10.1016/S1474-4422(20)30109-5.
122. Sedaghat S, Karimi N. Guillain Barre syndrome associated with COVID-19 infection: a case report. J Clin Neurosci. 2020;76:233–5.
123. Toscano G, Palmerini F, Ravaglia S, et al. Guillain-Barré syndrome associated with SARS-CoV-2. N Engl J Med. 2020;382(26):2574–6. https://doi.org/10.1056/NEJMc2009191.
124. Gutiérrez-Ortiz C, Méndez-Guerrero A, Rodrigo Rey S, et al. Miller fisher syndrome and polyneuritis cranialis in COVID-19. Neurology. 2020;95(5):e601–5. https://doi.org/10.1212/WNL.0000000000009619.
125. Kajani S, Kajani R, Huang CW, et al. Miller fisher syndrome in the COVID-19 era - a novel target antigen calls for novel treatment. Cureus. 2021;13(1):e12424. https://doi.org/10.7759/cureus.12424.
126. Cascella M, Del Gaudio A, Vittori A, Bimonte S, Del Prete P, Forte CA, Cuomo A, De Blasio E. COVID-Pain: Acute and Late-Onset Painful Clinical Manifestations in COVID-19 - Molecular Mechanisms and Research Perspectives. J Pain Res. 2021;14:2403–12. https://doi.org/10.2147/JPR.S313978.
127. Widyadharma IPE, Sari NNSP, Pradnyaswari KE, et al. Pain as clinical manifestations of COVID-19 infection and its management in the pandemic era: a literature review. Egypt J Neurol Psychiatr Neurosurg. 2020;56(1):121. https://doi.org/10.1186/s41983-020-00258-0.
128. Ali AM, Kunugi H. Skeletal muscle damage in COVID-19: a call for action. Medicina. 2021;57:372. https://doi.org/10.3390/medicina57040372.
129. Jin M, Tong Q. Rhabdomyolysis as potential late complication associated with COVID-19. Emerg Infect Dis. 2020;26(7):1618–20. https://doi.org/10.3201/eid2607.200445.
130. Pitscheider L, Karolyi M, Burkert FR, et al. Muscle involvement in SARS-CoV-2 infection. Eur J Neurol. 2020;30 https://doi.org/10.1111/ene.14564.
131. Dalakas MC. Inflammatory myopathies: update on diagnosis, pathogenesis and therapies, and COVID-19-related implications. Acta Myol. 2020;39(4):289–301. https://doi.org/10.36185/2532-1900-032.
132. Rogers JP, Chesney E, Oliver D, et al. Psychiatric and neuropsychiatric presentations associated with severe coronavirus infections: a systematic review and meta-analysis with comparison to the COVID-19 pandemic. Lancet Psychiatry. 2020;7:611–27.

133. Jasti M, Nalleballe C, Dandu V, et al. A review of pathophysiology and neuropsychiatric manifestations of COVID-19. Brain Behav Immun. 2020;88:71–4. https://doi.org/10.1016/j.bbi.2020.06.020.
134. Dubey S, Biswas P, Ghosh R, et al. Psychosocial impact of COVID-19. Diabetes Metab Syndr Clin Res Rev. 2020;14:779e788135.
135. Brooks SK, Webster RK, Smith LE, et al. The psychological impact of quarantine and how to reduce it: rapid review of the evidence. Lancet. 2020;395:912–20.
136. Lewnard JA, Lo NC. Scientific and ethical basis for social distancing interventions against COVID-19. Lancet Infect Dis. 2020;20(6):631–3. https://doi.org/10.1016/S1473-3099(20)30190-0.
137. Celis-Rodríguez E, Birchenall C, de la Cal MA, et al. Clinical practice guidelines for evidence-based management of sedoanalgesia in critically ill adult patients. Med Intensiva. 2013;37(8):519–74. https://doi.org/10.1016/j.medin.2013.04.001.
138. Vincent JL, Shehabi Y, Walsh TS, et al. Comfort and patient-centred care without excessive sedation: the eCASH concept. Intensive Care Med. 2016;42(6):962–71. https://doi.org/10.1007/s00134-016-4297-4.
139. Barr J, Fraser GL, Puntillo K, et al. Clinical practice guidelines for the management of pain, agitation, and delirium in adult patients in the intensive care unit. Crit Care Med. 2013;41(1):263–306. https://doi.org/10.1097/CCM.0b013e3182783b72.
140. Zhang H, Yuan J, Chen O, et al. Development and validation of a predictive score for ICU delirium in critically ill patients. BMC Anesthesiol. 2021;21(1):37. https://doi.org/10.1186/s12871-021-01259-z.
141. Devlin JW, Skrobik Y, Gélinas C, et al. Clinical practice guidelines for the prevention and management of pain, agitation/sedation, delirium, immobility and sleep disruption in adult patients in the ICU. Crit Care Med. 2018;46(9):e825–73. https://doi.org/10.1097/CCM.0000000000003299.
142. Garcez FB, Aliberti MJR, Poco PCE, et al. Delirium and adverse outcomes in hospitalized patients with COVID-19. J Am Geriatr Soc. 2020;68:2440–6. https://doi.org/10.1111/jgs.16803.
143. Ticinesi A, Cerundolo N, Parise A, et al. Delirium in COVID-19: epidemiology and clinical correlations in a large group of patients admitted to an academic hospital. Aging Clin Exp Res. 2020;32:2159–66.
144. Soysal P, Kara O. Delirium as the first clinical presentation of the coronavirus disease 2019 in an older adult. Psychogeriatrics. 2020;20(5):763–5. https://doi.org/10.1111/psyg.12587.
145. Tay HS, Harwood R. Atypical presentation of COVID-19 in a frail older person. Age Ageing. 2020;49(4):523–4. https://doi.org/10.1093/ageing/afaa068.
146. Helms J, Kremer S, Merdji H, et al. Delirium and encephalopathy in severe COVID-19: a cohort analysis of ICU patients. Crit Care. 2020;24:491.
147. Marra A, Ely EW, Pandharipande PP, Patel MB. The ABCDEF bundle in critical care. Crit Care Clin. 2017;33(2):225–43. https://doi.org/10.1016/j.ccc.2016.12.005.
148. Kotfis K, Roberson W, Wilson JE, et al. COVID-19: ICU delirium management during SARS-CoV-2 pandemic. Crit Care. 2020;24:176.
149. Pun BT, Badenes R, La Calle GH, et al. Prevalence and risk factors for delirium in critically ill patients with COVID-19 (COVID-D): a multicentre cohort study. Lancet Respir Med. 2021; S2213-2600(20)30552-X
150. Mistraletti G, Giannini A, Gristina G, et al. Why and how to open intensive care units to family visits during the pandemic. Crit Care. 2021;25:191. https://doi.org/10.1186/s13054-021-03608-3.

Diagnostic Approaches to Acute Neuro-COVID

3

3.1 Introduction

Although the pulmonary manifestations are the hallmark of COVID-19, there is increasing recognition of neurologic manifestations. To date, it has not been possible to clearly define the neuropathological picture underlying the disease and to identify which mechanisms are involved in the genesis of the nervous tissue damage. Various pathogenetic hypotheses have been formulated. They include direct SARS-CoV-2 neuroinvasion and endotheliopathy, indirect damage of the endothelium because of the release of cytokines, production of antibodies in the post-infectious phase, and systemic coagulopathy causing occlusion of cerebral vessels and/or bleeding [1–3]. Other potential effects include venous thrombosis and subarachnoid hemorrhage (SAH) [1, 4–6]. Furthermore, extracranial artery dissection has been also reported [7, 8]. Direct SARS-CoV-2 neuroinvasion could be the pathologic event leading to possible encephalitis or meningoencephalitis [9], while post-infection delayed immune response seems to be the cause of Guillain-Barre Syndrome (GBS) [10] and acute demyelinating encephalomyelitis [11]. Finally, complications could be related to systemic disease-related effects, such as severe hypoxia, or side effects of the therapy; extended hospitalization in the intensive care unit (ICU) with prolonged intubation may result in hypoxemic cerebral injury and microhemorrhages [9, 11–13]. More details can be found in another section of the book (see Chap. 1. Pathophysiology of COVID-19-associated neurotoxicity).

The neurological symptoms and signs are non-specific and often subtle, mainly in ICU sedated and ventilated patients. It is a challenging task for the clinician to differentiate between direct involvement of the central nervous system (CNS) and neurologic manifestations of systematic causes such as metabolic complications or hypoxia. All these conditions could delay the correct diagnosis and proper treatment.

Moreover, the enormous impact of the pandemic on the organizational system could make it difficult to obtain imaging studies and/or electrodiagnostic tests timely for the appropriate treatment. Therefore, a high index of clinical suspicion

M. Cascella, E. De Blasio, *Features and Management of Acute and Chronic Neuro-Covid*, https://doi.org/10.1007/978-3-030-86705-8_3

for neurological complications is required, and every effort should be done to reach early a definitive diagnosis to guide the therapy. In this contest, besides a complete clinical evaluation, it is necessary to submit these patients to a detailed neuroradiological, laboratory, and neurophysiological work-up.

3.2 Neuroimaging

Computer tomography (CT) and magnetic resonance imaging (MRI) are commonly used in COVID-19. These imaging approaches depicted several neuroradiological aspects because of the multiple pathological mechanisms involved [14].

3.2.1 Stroke

Thromboembolic infarcts are the most common neuroradiologic finding in COVID-19, accounting for 92% of patients who have an abnormal neuroimaging examination. Acute ischemic stroke mainly involves large vessels (60–65%), multiple vascular territories (26%), and vertebro-basilar territory (35%) [15]. It is a strong prognostic indicator of poor outcome [16].

The cerebral thromboembolic event may be the first presentation of COVID-19 and the episodes may coincide with increased D-dimer levels and inflammatory markers [17]. Several neuroimaging approaches can be used (Fig. 3.1):

- Non-contrast CT is the primary choice for the initial evaluation of patients suspected of stroke. Since CT is widely available, a scan can be made within a few minutes and unstable patients are easier to manage in a CT scanner than in an MRI one. Non-contrast CT provides enough information to quickly differentiate between ischemic and hemorrhagic stroke.
- CT-Angiography (CTA) can be performed in the case of acute stroke to detect or determine the location of thrombus, or occlusion. Large intracranial vessels such as the internal carotid artery and middle cerebral artery trunk can be excellently assessed using CTA for detecting occlusion.
- CT perfusion (CTP) is ideally suited for differentiating between the penumbra and the infarct core. In general, it holds that a decreased cerebral blood flow (CBF) value combined with a stable or increased cerebral blood volume (CBV), depicts reversible ischemia. On the other hand, a significant decrease of both CBF and CBV involves irreversible infarction.

An MRI examination requires more acquisition time, but according to the guideline, it should be considered more useful than a CT scan for diagnosing acute ischemic stroke. Diffusion-Weighted Imaging (DWI) offers the option of detecting parenchymal ischemia and/or an infarct within minutes from the occurrence of the first stroke symptoms. Perfusion MRI offers the potential for measuring brain perfusion in acute stroke patients. Arterial spin labeling (ASL) MR perfusion is an MRI

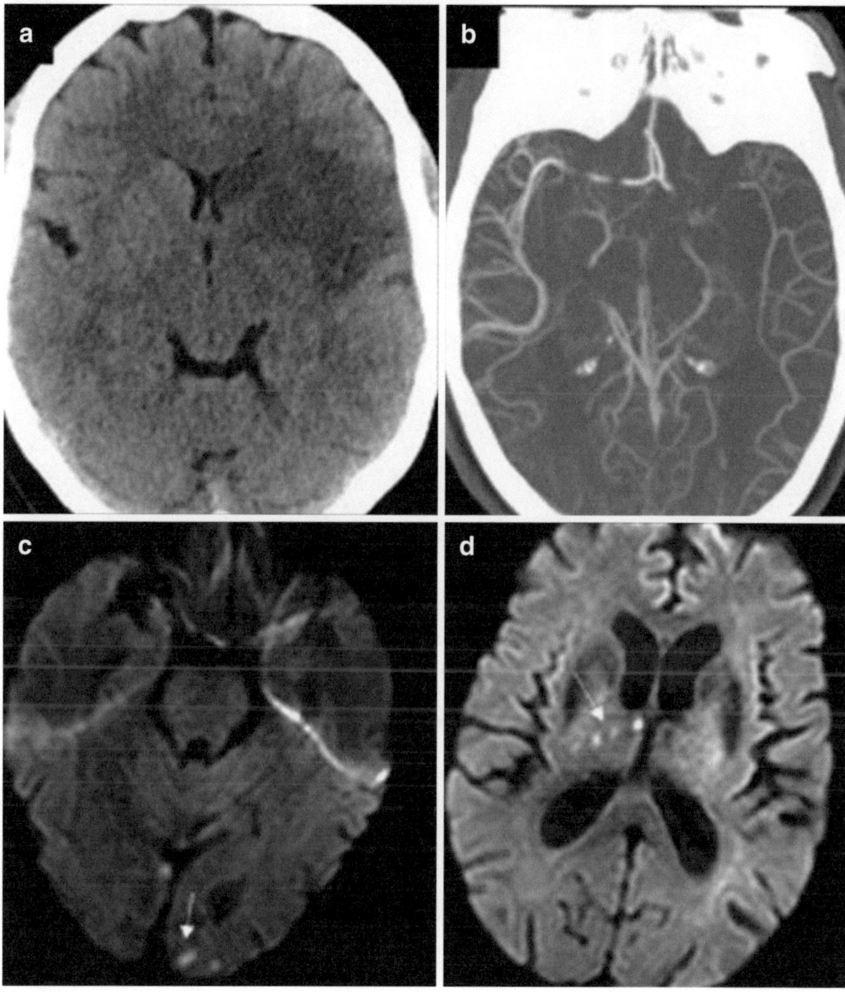

Fig. 3.1 Ischemic stroke. (**a**, **b**) Large vessel occlusion (non-contrast and contrast CT showing acute infarct in the left middle cerebral artery territory). (**c**, **d**) Embolic infarcts (MRI showing multiple punctate acute infarcts in multiple vascular territories). Modified from Agarwall A, et al. Emergency Radiology 2020(27);747–754 with permission

perfusion technique that does not require intravenous administration of contrast unlike dynamic susceptibility contrast (DSC) perfusion and dynamic contrast enhancement (DCE) perfusion.

Venous infarcts are uncommon. Cavalcanti et al. [18] reported three fatal cases of COVID-19 related to superficial and deep venous thrombosis. The diagnosis may require a brain MRI or a MR venography or CT venography to assess patency of the dural venous sinuses and cerebral veins. A method for 3D image reconstruction such as maximum intensity projection (MIP) can be helpful (Fig. 3.2).

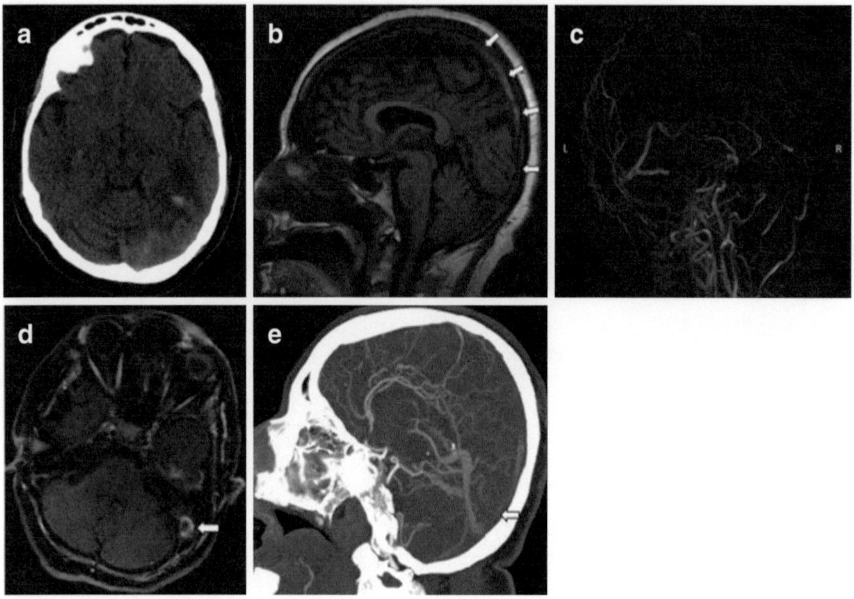

Fig. 3.2 Extensive venous sinus thrombosis. Axial CT Head demonstrated edema in the left temporal lobe with small parenchymal hemorrhage (**a**). Sag T1 on the MRI without contrast showed hyperintensity in superior sagittal sinus consistent with thrombus (arrows) (**b**). MR venogram maximum intensity projection (MIP) reconstruction demonstrated no flow in the superior sagittal sinus and left transverse sinus (**c**). Axial T1 sequence on MRI brain with contrast demonstrated this thrombus extending to the left jugular bulb (arrow) (**d**). Sagittal CT venography MIP reformat showed no flow in the superior sagittal sinus (arrow) (**e**). From Kihira S, et al. Clinical Imaging 69 (2021) 280–284 © Elsevier with permission

3.2.2 Cerebral Hemorrhagic Lesions

The cerebral hemorrhagic lesions account for 21.7%–25.7% of strokes and can be massive and/or multiple [15]. Patients may present with lobar hemorrhage, microhemorrhage, SAH, or subdural hemorrhage. Microhemorrhage occurred predominantly in the juxtacortical and callosal white matter. Several complications of COVID-19, such as disseminated intravascular coagulation caused by cytokine storm, blood pressure changes commonly occurring in the critical care setting. In these patients, anticoagulation therapy for venous thrombus prevention and acute kidney injury requiring dialysis [15] may contribute to intracranial hemorrhages.

The non-contrast head CT is the most commonly performed technique in the emergency evaluation. Additional diagnostic information may be obtained by CTA or MRI with contrast media. The neuroimaging must evaluate location, size/volume, shape (irregular/regular), density (homogeneous/heterogeneous), and presence/absence of substantial surrounding edema (underlying tumor), intraventricular hemorrhage, or hydrocephalus. The ABC/2 formula or more accurate tools (e.g., 2.5ABC/6, SH/2) can help for the analyses.

3.2.3 Mixed Pictures

The various vascular manifestations could be seen simultaneously in a single patient. In fact, in the first case reported, Dorigatti et al. [19] described a patient with a wide range of vascular findings at brain MRI. After weaning from sedation and ventilation, a 67-year-old man with severe respiratory distress syndrome appeared with spontaneous eye opening although unresponsive to the verbal, tactile, and painful stimulus; no focal deficits were found. The MRI showed cortico-subcortical and callosal microbleeds, SAH, intraparenchymal hematoma, and reduced CBF in the frontoparietal regions juxtaposed to the vascular border zones, as seen at both ASL and DSC perfusion techniques. The authors supposed that multiple pathological mechanisms could lead to the described findings. Among these mechanisms, hypoxemia and blood–brain barrier (BBB) disruption were discussed. The importance of the use of a non-invasive ASL technique, that could allow the study of CBF and its correlation with the prognostic outcome, was addressed.

In a retrospective review on 103 COVID-19 patients submitted to neuroimaging (MRI, CT, or CTA) for mild non-focal neurological symptoms, such as headache, transient ataxia, mild confusion, and dysarthria, normal findings were found in most subjects (74.7%) (all the patients with seizures or post-sedation encephalopathy); among the others, there was a large variation of the incidence of positive neuroimaging findings (from 10% in patients with mild non-focal symptoms to 68% of patients with suspected stroke/TIA). The authors did not find specific neuroimaging presentations. Probably, multifactorial causes, such as coagulopathy and immuno-mediated para-infectious mechanisms (cytokine storm), were at the basis of these findings [20]. Other factors, such as critical illness-related encephalopathy, and withdrawal of medications could be involved.

Nevertheless, some reports showed a higher incidence of positive findings. In a report on 58 ICU patients with unexplained encephalopathic features, such as agitation, dysexecutive syndrome, and corticospinal signs, the MRI was performed in 13 patients. Bilateral frontotemporal hypoperfusion was noted in all 11 patients who underwent perfusion imaging, while enhancement in leptomeningeal spaces was found in 8, and small ischemic stroke in 3 patients. Even in this study, it was difficult to demonstrate a correlation between neuroimaging findings and specific neuropathogenic mechanisms [21].

A case series of COVID-19 critically ill patients with CNS involvement reported the results of neuroimaging studies in patients with focal signs of acute ischemic stroke at the presentation, status epilepticus, and delayed/negative wake-up at the end of sedation. The CT study showed a lacunar ischemic stroke in 25% of the cases. Follow-up MRI showed multiple bilateral early subacute ischemic lesions in different vascular territories, expression of small-vessel disease. No acute findings at CT and MRI were found in patients experiencing status epilepticus. Among the patients with delayed wake-up at the end of sedation, the neuroimaging showed multiple cerebral microbleeds, with SAH in 3 cases, and additional small ischemic lesions in 2 cases. The CT or MR angiographic studies performed in 7 patients showed no signs of vasculitis. Of note, intracranial vessel wall sequence MRI was performed in 3 patients. It showed contrast enhancement of vessel walls in large cerebral arteries, suggesting an inflammatory component of the vascular wall; this finding was interpreted as unspecific endothelial dysfunction. Based on these findings, the authors concluded that, besides early acute ischemic stroke, a small cerebral vessel involvement can occur later. As suggested by microinfarctions and vessel wall contrast enhancement, the inflammatory vascular wall damage was postulated to be the underlying mechanisms [22].

The involvement of small vessels was also described in a 65-year-old man with severe respiratory failure who was unarousable after the discontinuation of sedation. The CT study showed multiple white matter, basal ganglia, and cerebellar ischemic hypodensities, as well as bilateral globus pallidus hyperdensities, suggestive of hemorrhage. The MRI confirmed the extensive ischemic lesions with restricted diffusion, involving the centrum semiovale, corpus callosum, basal ganglia, and cerebellum with patchy/punctuate enhancement without abnormalities of large intra and extracranial arteries. In this case, the authors hypothesized involvement of the small intracranial vessels with a vasculitis-like pattern [23].

In COVID-19 patients, the increased risk of developing microvascular lesions was confirmed in an MRI study in mechanically ventilated patients because of acute respiratory distress syndrome (ARDS). These patients were unresponsive and/or with focal neurologic deficits. The susceptibility weighted imaging (SWI) MRI showed punctate foci of abnormal susceptibility signal, in 69% of cases with over 10 lesions in 50% of those; multiple clustered lesions involved the corpus callosum were found in 25%. In subjects with multiple lesions, alterations were detected in subcortical and deep white matter, with variable involvement of the brainstem, and cerebellum. Notably, a brain autopsy showed mixed microhemorrhages and microscopic ischemic lesions; the hemorrhagic lesions were identified with SWI, while the small size of ischemic lesions prevented their detection with MRI. These aspects may suggest that cerebral microvascular lesions, both hemorrhagic and ischemic, are common findings in severe COVID-19 patients with neurologic deficits although the ischemic lesions could be difficult to identify [24].

3.2.4 Posterior Reversible Encephalopathy Syndrome

Posterior reversible encephalopathy syndrome (PRES) has been described in patients with COVID-19 [25]. It is characterized by clinical and neuroradiological findings caused by vasogenic edema linked to alteration of cerebrovascular autoregulation (Fig. 3.3).

The first report concerned two patients with acute kidney failure and moderate hypertension [25]. The clinical picture was characterized by altered consciousness during the weaning from mechanical ventilation. MRI showed T2 fluid-attenuated inversion recovery (FLAIR) hyperintensity signal involving the subcortical white matter of occipital lobes and/or posterior temporal lobes and cerebellar hemisphere, with effacement of the adjacent sulci. Axial SWI showed convexal subarachnoid hemorrhage in a case, and petechial hemorrhage, in the other one. DWI and

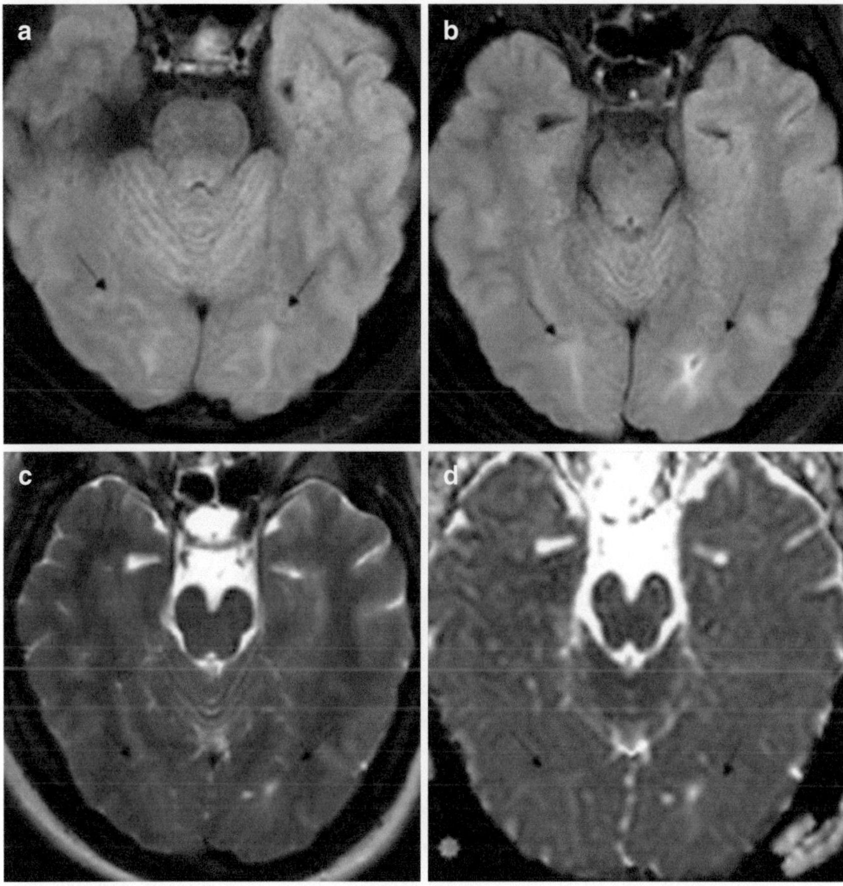

Fig. 3.3 Posterior reversible encephalopathy syndrome. Axial T2-FLAIR images (**a, b**) and axial T2-spine echo image (**c**): near-symmetric areas of subcortical signal changes with edema and sulcal effacement in the occipital lobes. Apparent diffusion coefficient (ADC) maps (**d**): increased signal representing facilitated diffusion as seen in vasogenic edema. From Agarwall A, et al. Emergency Radiology 2020(27);747–754 with permission

T1-weighted images after administration of gadolinium were unremarkable. The patients were treated with antihypertensives with a gradual recovery of symptomatology. About mechanisms, it can be hypnotized that, in COVID-19, the endothelial dysfunction could induce PRES at lower levels of blood pressure. Consequently, stricter control of blood pressure is required [25].

In another case report, neuroimaging features showed vasogenic edema. These features were predominant in the parieto-occipital lobes but also in frontal, and cerebellar regions, basal ganglia, as well as in corpus callosum, and in some cases parenchymal hemorrhages, and SHA. The authors underlined the importance of early detection of neurological symptomatology to submit the patients to MRI studies, either in the acute phase or during the follow-up to determine the radiologic outcomes [26]. Other four cases of PRES were reported from the United States (US). Acute kidney injury and elevated blood pressure were present in all of these patients. The encephalopathic and epileptiform activity were reported in two cases. CT findings were characterized by bilateral hypoattenuation involving the bilateral occipital or parieto-occipital white matter, confirmed by MRI. It showed confluent T2 hyperintensities, without ischemic diffusion restriction on DWI or susceptibility hypointensity, *associated* with the presence of symptomatic *hemorrhage* in the same regions. In one patient, diffusion restriction reflecting cytotoxic edema and indicating ischemia was demonstrated. The authors postulated that the cytokine storm could increase vascular permeability; upregulation of vascular endothelial growth factor in the setting of hypoxia leading to vasogenic edema was also suggested. In this setting, the use of some drugs for the treatment of SARS-CoV-2 infection, such as tocilizumab and hydroxychloroquine, could play a role in the pathogenesis of PRES [27]. Another case series of four patients with agitation and spatial disorientation and one case with generalized seizure after weaning from mechanical ventilation, the MRI study showed multiple areas, from punctiform to some millimeters in extension, hyperintense on T2-weighted and FLAIR images, located in the parietal, occipital, and frontal regions. On DWI, all but two lesions were characterized by the absence of apparent diffusion coefficient (ADC) changes related to acute ischemic events. There was a minimum involvement of the adjacent subcortical white matter in only a few lesions, while SWI sequences did not show alterations. In addition, a subtle contrast enhancement was detected only in a cortical lesion. Based on the prevalent cortical involvement and DWI pattern (not typical of this syndrome), the authors hypothesized a multifactorial mechanism that encompassed such as vasomotor reactivity dysregulation, with transient vasoconstriction, endothelial dysfunction, and impaired microcirculation [28].

Finally, some atypical presentations of PRES have been also described in the literature. In particular, MRI was characterized by areas of vasogenic edema, predominantly in parieto-occipital regions, associated with diffuse petechiae or intraparenchymal hematoma. Probably, the combined action of the massive cytokine release with a breakdown of the BBB, and coagulation impairment are involved in the pathogenic cascade [29, 30].

3.2.5 Encephalitis

Scientific evidence on encephalitis due to SARS-CoV-2 is sparse and based on case reports. In the first case described in the literature, a patient presenting with unconsciousness, seizures, fever, and neck stiffness following the respiratory symptoms of SARS-CoV-2 was submitted to brain MRI after the ICU admission. A diagnosis of right lateral ventriculitis and encephalitis was made based on the following findings: (i) DWI hyperintensity along the wall of the inferior horn of right lateral ventricle; (ii) FLAIR images showing hyperintense signal changes in the right mesial temporal lobe and hippocampus with slight hippocampal atrophy; (iii) no definite dural enhancement with contrast-enhanced imaging [31]. In other case reports, neuroimaging studies were not performed or did not find pathological evidence at CT or MRI, even in presence of pathological CSF findings [32–35].

In a retrospective single-center study on 222 COVID-19 patients, encephalitis was described in 9.5% of patients, while acute meningitis was found in 1.4%. Among the patients with suspected encephalitis, brain MRI was performed in all the 22 patients with confirmed/probable encephalitis. The results were highly heterogeneous showing unifocal/multifocal ischemic lesions, small vessel infarcts, and microhemorrhages. Other lesions were basal ganglia FLAIR hyperintensity, acute diffuse hemispheric white matter lesions, FLAIR hyperintensity of the genu of the corpus callosum, mesiotemporal FLAIR hyperintensity with fronto-insular extension, brainstem, and cerebellar peduncular FLAIR hyperintensity, cranial nerve FLAIR hyperintensity, and focal leptomeningeal FLAIR hyperintensity [36].

Some acute severe forms of demyelinating encephalitis could affect COVID-19 patients. In a patient with a decreased level of consciousness and no focal deficits and seizures at EEG, the MRI revealed hyperintensities in T2WI of the periventricular white matter, without restriction of diffusion on DWI nor contrast enhancement on T1-weighted images. Similar lesions were found at the bulbo-medullary junction, and in both the cervical and dorsal spinal cord [37]. Similarly, in a patient with a wake-up delay after sedation and intubation, brain CT showed hypodense lesions involving supratentorial white matter and pallidum bilaterally. In this patient, the MRI demonstrated acute ischemic lesions on DWI without any hemorrhage or enhancement after gadolinium injection and sparing of the thalamus, striatum, and the posterior fossa. Based on the bilateral and asymmetrical lesions in the deep layers of the white matter, acute demyelination can be hypothesized [38].

A patient with coma and impaired oculocephalic response to one side was submitted to an MRI study after 24 days from the onset of the respiratory symptomatology. The neuroimaging showed scattered hyperintense lesions on FLAIR imaging in deep hemispheric, and juxtacortical white matter. These lesions were not consistent with acute ischemic lesions on DWI. A FLAIR hyperintensity lesion in the left frontal juxtacortical white matter showed mild enhancement with gadolinium contrast. A small intraventricular hemorrhage was seen in the occipital horns of both lateral ventricles. The gradient-echo sequence did not show evidence of parenchymal hemorrhage. The patient was diagnosed with acute disseminated encephalomyelitis (ADEM) and was treated with steroids and intravenous immunoglobulin with an improvement of symptomatology. The MRI follow-up showed an increase in the number and distribution of FLAIR-T2 hyperintense lesions, and a new-onset right frontal enhancing lesion [39].

In the literature, sporadic cases of acute hemorrhagic leukoencephalitis (AHLE) which is a subtype of ADEM are reported. Five weeks after a SARS-CoV-2 infection, a patient showed headache, altered mental status, and loss of left limb power. The initial MRI scan showed white matter multifocal asymmetric lesions that increased in number and size with intralesional hemorrhage leading to edema, transtentorial herniation, vascular compression, infarcts in bilateral posterior cerebral artery territories. In particular, typical neuroimaging features of AHLE are multifocal, variable-sized (often over 1 cm), poorly defined white matter lesions involving both cerebral hemispheres but predominantly in the parietal and occipital lobes with the characteristic asymmetric distribution. A less frequent involvement was described for the brainstem, cerebellar peduncle, and deep gray matter. The lesions appear hyperintense on T2 fast spin echo (FSE) and FLAIR weighted images, and hypointense on T1-weighted images; they can also show microhemorrhage-related blooming in SWI. The DWI and T1-weighted contrast enhancement characteristics are quite variable. On these bases, the importance of the differential diagnosis of ADEM/AHLE from other forms of encephalitis is mandatory. The ADEM is characterized by multiple, asymmetric, poorly marginated lesions, smaller in size, with less severe edema, and additional spinal cord involvement, without hemorrhage and enhancement. On the other hand, ANE findings display characteristic symmetric signal changes with thalamic involvement, and additional lesions at the level of the brainstem, cerebral white matter, and cerebellum [40].

Another issue concerns acute necrotizing encephalopathy (ANE). This severe type of encephalitis develops by various viral infections (e.g., influenza A and B, herpesvirus, varicella, and rotavirus), and affects predominantly the children. Probably, the underlying pathogenetic mechanism involves the combination of systemic cytokine storm (without vessel disruption) with viral invasion, and para-infectious demyelination. A case report described a patient with a history of fever, cough, and altered mental status. Unenhanced brain CT demonstrated symmetric low attenuation within the bilateral medial thalami with normal CT angiogram and venogram. Brain MRI showed hemorrhagic rim-enhancing lesions within the bilateral thalami, medial temporal lobes, and subinsular regions. The pathological mechanism was ascribed to intracranial cytokine storm or para-infectious demyelination [41].

From the data reported in the literature, it emerges that a precise characterization of neurological lesions and neuroimaging correlates is an extremely difficult task. However, neurological damages are not that rare how they look. A larger retrospective analysis (n = 167) in patients with neurological signs or symptoms such as delirium, altered level of consciousness, and focal neurologic signs, confirmed the wide range of abnormal neuroimaging findings. The most common finding at CT was subacute infarct (44.4%), followed by acute infarct (38.9%), and less frequently basal ganglia hemorrhage (11.1%), and SAH (5.6%). Most patients presenting with altered consciousness and delirium were investigated with MRI. Callosal or parenchymal/callosal microhemorrhages were present in 60% of patients. Watershed white matter hyperintensities on T2 FLAIR images (cerebral deep watershed areas, corpus callosum, and cerebellar white matter) were found in 20% of patients with microhemorrhages. On SWI, these findings were seen in superficial veins with microhemorrhages, in 15% of patients, acute infarcts in 15%, and subacute infarcts, in 10% of patients. Other findings on MRI were acute hemorrhagic necrotizing encephalopathy with bilateral cortical, and subcortical lesions in parieto-occipital lobes, with the appearance of PRES-like pattern (10%), large parenchymal hemorrhage (10%), and less frequently, hypoxic changes, SAH, and ADEM-like changes (5%). The wide spectrum of neuroimaging findings can be explained by multiple pathogenetic mechanisms involved in the cerebral damage. These mechanisms can include endothelial dysfunction, systemic hypoxemia, hypercoagulable state with formation of microthrombi, and cytotoxic and vasogenic edema [42].

3.2.6 Myelitis

An increasing number of cases of myelitis have been reported in the literature. Myelitis can be clinically expressed in terms of motor symptoms (until complete plegia), sensitive symptomatology, and sphincter dysfunction. Transverse myelitis is the most common syndrome, followed by partial transverse myelitis, Brown Sequard syndrome, and dorsal columns syndrome [43–47]. MRI has been used as an imaging modality of choice in the differential diagnosis, ruling out other conditions with similar symptomatology. In a patient with spastic paraparesis, MRI demonstrated multifocal transverse myelitis with a patchy hyperintensity of the thoracic myelon at Th9–10 and at Th3–5 level [43]. In another patient with sudden onset paraplegia and urinary retention, a gadolinium-enhanced MRI demonstrated an extensive diffuse hyperintense signal in T2-weighted images. This finding concerned especially the gray matter of the cervical, dorsal, and lumbar spinal cord; mild enlargement and swelling of the cervical cord but no spinal cord or nerve root enhancement and hemorrhagic components was found; furthermore, DWI showed areas of restricted diffusion (Fig. 3.4) [44].

Canavero et al. [45] reported three cases of acute myelopathies with different MRI findings at brain and spine; the first patient showed multifocal cervical lesions,

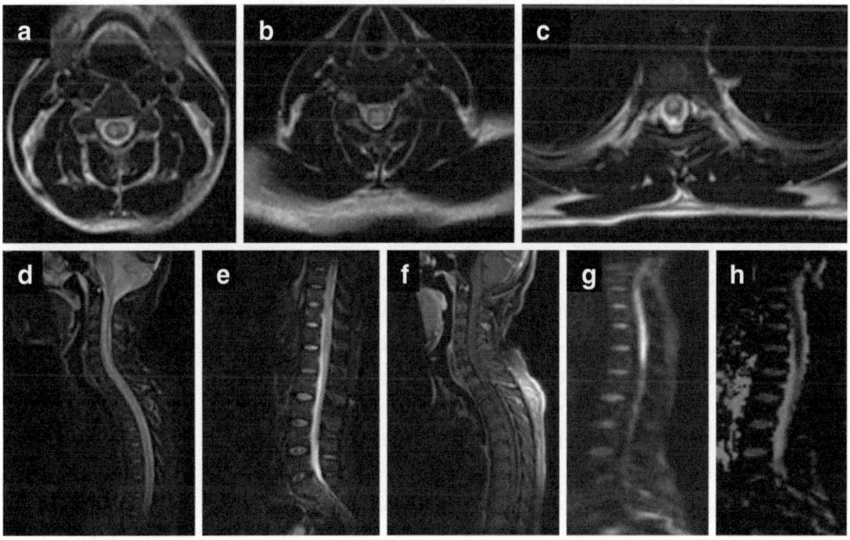

Fig. 3.4 Acute myelitis. (**a–c**) axial T2 images of cervical and dorsal spine showing central hyperintense signal of the cervical and dorsal spinal cord. (**d**, **e**) sagittal short tau inversion recovery (STIR) images of cervical, dorsal, and lumbar spine showing hyperintense longitudinal signal involving a long segment of the spinal cord starting at the level of C2. (**f**) T1 Gadolinium enhanced MRI of cervical and upper dorsal spine in sagittal view showing no evidence of abnormal enhancement of the spinal cord. (**g**, **h**) diffusion-weighted imaging (DWI) and apparent diffusion coefficient (ADC) sagittal images showing evidence of restricted diffusion. From AlKetbi et al., Radiology Case Reports 15 (2020) 1591–1595 © Elsevier with permission

mainly involving the cervical lateral and dorsal centro-medullary region with normal brain findings; the second had diffuse hyperintensity in T2-weighted images from bulbo-medullary junction to C6 and conus with central sparing and a single right posterior periventricular lesion; the third patient presented with multiple lesions at the cervical and upper thoracic spinal level and with a longitudinal elongated transverse myelitis (LETM) from mid-thoracic to the epiconus with preeminent involvement of the anterior horns. In the latter case, MRI showed a single lesion in the left superior cerebellar peduncle. As the authors stated, multiple pathologic mechanisms, such as direct viral pathogenicity, immune-mediated damage, inflammatory vascular processes, and intravascular coagulation can be involved [45]. Of note, it seems that MRI findings of COVID-19-associated myelitis did not show differences from those of non-COVID-19 patients. Findings such as isolated or multifocal hyperintense lesions on STIR or T2-weighted MRI images in the cervical and thoracic cord, sometimes accompanied by tissue edema and enlargement of the spinal cord, are not exclusive of COVID-19. Moreover, there was no pathological gadolinium enhancement, while the evidence of restricted diffusion on DWI sequences indicated cytotoxic edema that can be found in many pathological pictures [46]. Thus, clinical and radiological characteristics of COVID-19 para-infectious myelitis are variable and non-specific. Nevertheless, since myelitis can affect COVID-19 patients with a different degree of disease (from asymptomatic to more serious cases), a prompt diagnosis could be very challenging [47].

3.2.7 Peripheral Nervous System and Muscular Disorders

Imaging studies could be helpful in the differential diagnosis of the peripheral nervous system (PNS) and muscular disorders. In COVID-19 patients with peripheral nerve injuries, indications, and differences of the various techniques have been highlighted. The High-Spatial-Resolution US is easy to perform and can be helpful to monitor the evolution of the lesions, even in more critical patients. Its portability is helpful as it avoids transporting the patients and, in turn, the need of disinfecting the radiological suite. On the other hand, MRI allows a large field-of-view assessment of the muscles and avoids problems of acoustic windows, and the prolonged close contact of the physician during the procedure [48].

MRI findings of GBS and its variants include signal hyperintensity, enlargement, and mild-to-moderate contrast enhancement of the nerve roots/plexus, and cauda equina; in chronic inflammatory demyelinating polyneuropathy, contrast enhancement is usually not present [49]. In a case series of five patients with GBS, MRI showed on T1-weighted images enhancement of the caudal nerve roots, in two patients, enhancement of the facial nerve, in one patient, and no signal changes in nerves, in two patients [50]. In a case report of a Miller Fisher Syndrome (MFS), MRI with gadolinium of the brain, orbits, and retro-orbital regions showed a striking enlargement, prominent enhancement with gadolinium, and hyperintense signal on T2-weighted images of the left cranial nerve III, with no other abnormal findings of other cranial nerves, brain, and cerebellum [51]. Moreover, a systematic analysis on MRI study of the brain and cranial nerves showed abnormal enhancement of the III, VI, and VII cranial nerves in 35%. Leptomeningeal enhancement of the brainstem and cervical spine was found in one case. When the MRI examination of the lumbosacral spine was performed, abnormal spine nerve root enhancement was found in 27% [52]. In another systematic review of 73 cases of GBS and its variants, brain and spinal MRI (performed only in one-third of cases) showed cranial nerve contrast enhancement in five patients (AIDP, MFS, bilateral facial palsy with paresthesia) and brainstem leptomeningeal enhancement in two cases. Spinal nerve roots enhancement on T1-weighted images in eight cases and leptomeningeal enhancement in the other two cases were reported [53].

Chronic inflammatory demyelinating polyneuropathy has been reported as focal or diffuse enlargement, and signal hyperintensity of the peripheral nerves, nerve roots and/or plexus, and cauda equina, without contrast enhancement [48]. Other causes of peripheral nerve injuries could be the position-related injury, as after prone position, involving mainly radial, median, and common peroneal nerves. In these cases, the MRI has shown nerve signal hyperintensity, thickening, and fascicular enlargement; the ultrasound findings were nerve hypoechogenicity, thickening, and fascicular enlargement. The critical illness polyneuropathy, a complication of prolonged ICU stay, appears at MRI with diffuse symmetric nerve signal hyperintensity on T2-weighted images [48, 49].

Ultrasound, CT and MRI studies could identify also musculoskeletal and soft tissue complications of the SARS-CoV-2 infection. In cases of suspected myositis and rhabdomyolysis, MRI represents the exam of choice. It shows increased signal intensity on T2-weighted or short tau inversion recovery (STIR) sequences that express muscle edema. In cases of myonecrosis, areas of loss of normal architecture may be seen with a distinguishing finding of the "stipple sign" with foci of enhancement in a rim-enhancing area of non-enhancing muscle tissue. Areas of intramuscular hemorrhage may be identified as T1 hyperintense signal or blooming artifact on GE sequences. A differential diagnosis with critical illness myopathy can be made. The latter, indeed, appears with multifocal edema and atrophy without areas of necrosis [49]. In patients with back or leg pain, lower-extremity weakness, or lower-extremity paresthesia who underwent MRI, 78% had evidence of paraspinal myositis with intramuscular edema, manifested by T2 hyperintensity, and/or enhancement within the paraspinal muscles in the lumbar spine, involving bilaterally multiple vertebral body levels [54]. Furthermore, a case report described a COVID-19 patient with diffuse myalgia, proximal lower-limb muscle weakness, and elevated creatine kinase. Edema of the right vastus medialis at proximal (lower-limb MRI in T2 STIR sequence) and bilateral edema of external obturator muscles (pelvic MRI in T2 STIR sequence), as well as enhancement of muscle lesions after gadolinium infusion (T1 sequences), lead to the diagnosis of myositis [55]. Ultrasound studies can be helpful in the diagnosis of diaphragm dysfunction, showing a reduced thickness and excursion of the muscle. The same studies, performed through high-resolution ultrasound examination of the phrenic nerve at the level of the neck, could help to identify the neuropathic or myopathic cause of diaphragm dysfunction [49]. MRI performed in critical illness myopathy in patients with a prolonged hospital stay showed multifocal intramuscular edema-like signal setting, and fatty infiltration and atrophy, respectively, in the acute and the chronic phase [48, 49].

3.2.8 Clinical and Neuroimaging Correlation

Given the wide range of clinical and radiological findings and the growing number of reports, it could be useful to correlate the clinical features to the neuroimaging findings. The aim is to summarize clinical and radiological findings in a comprehensive framework, identifying specific pictures. Furthermore, knowledge of underlying pathophysiological mechanisms could aid in diagnosis and treatment.

In COVID-19 ICU patients, Scullen et al. [56] found 35.5% of encephalopathies or cerebrovascular disease. They identified three clinical-radiological pictures:

- COVID-19-associated encephalopathy (74%).
- COVID-19-associated vasculopathy (19%).
- COVID-19-associated acute necrotizing encephalopathy (7%).

The most common CT findings included subacute ischemic strokes, diffuse hypoattenuation, subcortical parenchymal hemorrhages, and focal hypodensities in deep structures. Typical MRI findings were DWI, and FLAIR changes with bilateral diffuse involvement of the deep white matter, corpus callosum, and basal ganglia [56].

The wide range of CNS and PNS manifestations was confirmed in other analyses [57]. Based on the clinical, imaging, and laboratory features, the patients can be divided into five groups (Table 3.1):

Table 3.1 Clinical, imaging, and laboratory features of CNS and PNS manifestations [57]

Group	Clinic	Neuroimaging	Treatment
Encephalopathies	Delirium or psychosis	MRI: No specific changes	Supportive
Neuroinflammatory syndromes	Inflammatory syndromes with a reduced level of consciousness and abnormal upper motor neuron signs	MRI: Multifocal areas of signal change, multiple microhemorrhages and restricted diffusion and peripheral rim enhancement	Corticosteroids or corticosteroids/IVIG
Stroke	Vary because of the arterial territories	Vary because of the arterial territories	LMWE, aspirin and DOACs
Diseases of the peripheral nervous system[a]	Motor/sensory symptoms	Vary	IVIG/corticosteroids
Miscellaneous[b]	Vary	Vary	Vary

Abbreviations: *MRI* magnetic resonance imaging, *LMWE* low-molecular-weight heparin, *DOACs* direct oral anticoagulants, *IVIG* intravenous immunoglobulin
[a]For example, Guillain-Barre syndrome
[b]Disorders difficult to categorize and submitted to specific treatments

According to this approach, MRI has a key role to confirm or exclude the diagnosis, especially in ICU patients. It can guide therapy, balancing the risk and benefits of the treatments [57].

Another nosographic approach focused on eight neuroradiological patterns. Notably, ischemic/thrombotic lesions were not addressed [58]:

- Unilateral hyperintensities located in the medial temporal lobe on FLAIR or diffusion-weighted images (found in 43%).
- Nonconfluent multifocal white matter hyperintense lesions with variable enhancement on FLAIR and diffusion-weighted images (30%).
- Extensive and isolated white matter microhemorrhages (24%).
- Extensive and confluent supratentorial white matter hyperintensities on FLAIR images (11%).
- Hyperintense lesion located in the central part of the splenium of the corpus callosum on FLAIR, and diffusion-weighted images (5%).
- Nonconfluent multifocal white matter hyperintense lesions with variable enhancement associated with hemorrhagic lesions on FLAIR, and diffusion-weighted images (5%).
- ANE pictures. Symmetric thalamic lesions (edema, petechial hemorrhage, and necrosis), with variable involvement of the brainstem, internal capsule, putamen, cerebral, and cerebellar white matter (5%).
- Hyperintense lesions involving both middle cerebellar peduncles on FLAIR images (5%).

In about one-quarter of cases, the MRI showed two or three patterns. Furthermore, the presence of hemorrhage was associated with a worse clinical picture. It was hypothesized that in patients with severe COVID-19, the heterogeneity of MRI findings found could be explained by the heterogeneity of the pathogenetic mechanisms. Direct viral infection, vasculitis, immunological para-infectious process, post-infectious demyelinating disease, and metabolic hypoxic manifestation can be involved [58].

Other authors offered a more detailed classification [59]. In critically ill COVID-19 patients, they subdivided the neuroimaging findings in the following pictures:

- Acute ischemic stroke and vasculitis-like pattern.
- Cerebral venous thrombosis.
- Critically illness-associated cerebral microbleeds seen in blood-sensitive T2 gradient series.
- Hypertensive PRES, and in some cases hemorrhagic PRES.
- Leukoencephalopathy with microhemorrhagic changes (diffuse confluent posterior predominant white matter T2/FLAIR hyperintensities, and scattered microhemorrhages, without diffusion restriction).

- Hemodynamic hypoperfusion-hypoxic patterns, including watershed infarcts, hypoxic/ischemic encephalopathy, and delayed post-hypoxic leukoencephalopathy .
- Meningoencephalitis and flare-up of other infections:
  - Medial temporal and hippocampal involvement (abnormal bright T 2 signal involving the hippocampus).
  - Hemorrhagic necrotizing encephalitis.
  - Acute necrotizing encephalopathy.
- Acute disseminated encephalomyelitis.
- Spine manifestations, such as GBS.

An overview of neuroimaging findings of patients with COVID-2019 presenting with neurological manifestations was conducted by Chen et al. [60]. In this systematic review, the pooled proportion of abnormal findings in patients with neurological manifestations was 59%, 68% on MRI, and 46% on CT [60]. The main findings were as follows:

- Acute/subacute ischemic lesions on brain CT/MRI (22% of patients). Large and small vessels were involved, mainly the anterior circulatory artery (69.2% of cases). Of note, small cortical ischemic lesions were found on MRI studies even in absence of interstitial lung involvement or without an increase of systemic inflammatory markers.
- Intracranial hemorrhage on CT/MRI (24%). Microhemorrhages were visualized by SWI, presenting as hypoattenuating foci, mainly in ICU patients. Some unusual distributions were found in the corpus callosum, internal capsule, and middle cerebellar peduncles; macrohemorrhages were also observed with CT and MRI.
- White matter abnormalities (27%). FLAIR hyperintensities, and abnormal restricted diffusion in the corpus callosum, subcortical, deep white matter, cerebellar peduncles, and corticospinal tracts.
- Other findings. Leptomeningeal enhancement (post-contrast T1W1 or FLAIR images and better visualized by delayed post-contrast FLAIR), cortical abnormalities (increased FLAIR and diffusion-weighted signal with non-specific distribution), smaller olfactory bulb, and abnormal enhancement of oculomotor, abducens, and facial nerves. Most of these findings were associated with non-specific neurological symptoms, such as agitation, spatial disorientation, and weakness.

The high incidence of abnormal neuroimaging findings (42.6%) on brain CT or MRI was also confirmed by a systematic review and meta-analysis on 21 studies and 2125 patients. Acute/subacute infarcts were the most common finding (24%), followed by cerebral microhemorrhages (6.9%), acute spontaneous intracerebral hemorrhages (5.4%), and encephalitis/encephalopathy (3.3%). Moreover, a subgroup analysis has highlighted a significant higher pooled incidence of cerebral microhemorrhages (11.8%; $p < 0.001$) and encephalitis/encephalopathy (11.1%; $p < 0.001$) in ICU patients [61].

The association between abnormal findings and the severity of COVID-19 can be strictly related to the inflammatory state and the neurotropism of SARS-CoV-2. The endothelial damage due to a systemic vasculitis, and hypercoagulable state could lead to cerebrovascular complications, either ischemic or hemorrhagic. Similarly, the vasogenic subcortical edema in the posterior territories seen in PRES, with a higher prevalence of hemorrhagic subtype, could be linked to a massive release of cytokines with BBB damage. MRI findings of ADEM and ANE could be produced by the inflammatory changes, while the multifocal leukoencephalopathy could be an expression of demyelination or small-vessel vasculitis. Finally, some MRI abnormalities of the olfactory bulbs and tracts, orbital-frontal and gyrus rectus cortex, brain stem, thalami, hypothalamus, and medial temporal lobes could suggest a direct involvement of neural cells due to SARS-CoV-2 neurotropism [62].

At the MRI neuroimaging, acute/subacute infarction can be attributable to endothelial dysfunction, inflammation, or platelet dysfunction. Moreover, diffuse white matter abnormality is often combined with parenchymal microhemorrhages. These abnormalities can be ascribed to the systemic inflammation, leading to hypercoagulability and vascular endothelial damage, resulting in thrombotic microangiopathy. Leptomeningeal contrast enhancement is an expression of leptomeningitis. Furthermore, cortical T2 FLAIR hyperintense signal is an expression of different clinical conditions, such as encephalitis, postictal state, PRES, and acute ischemia. Based on these findings, it could be advisable to perform an MRI investigation in patients with mild and moderate symptomatology and not only in the most urgent cases. This strategy could be useful to determine the full spectrum of the CNS involvement, and understand the pathological mechanisms underlying the clinical manifestations [63].

3.2.9 The Role of Brain Positron Emission Tomography

Neuropsychiatric problems have been increasingly described in COVID-19 patients. Many of these cases are attributable to encephalitis that often are characterized by normal, or non-specific, CT, and MRI findings. Thus, other kinds of imaging stud ies, such as brain positron emission tomography (PET)/TC, could help to guide clinical management. A case of suspected autoimmune encephalitis has been reported in a patient showing symptoms signs of cerebellar syndrome, with tremor, ataxia, dysarthria, upper-limb dysmetria, and diffuse myoclonus. The electroencephalography (EEG) showed symmetric diffuse background slowing, reactive to stimulation, without interictal paroxysms, while the contrast-enhanced brain MRI was normal. The immunologic study revealed high titers of IgG autoantibodies in serum and CSF directed against the nuclei of Purkinje cells, striatal neurons, and hippocampal neurons. Brain PET with ^{18}F-fluorodeoxyglucose (^{18}F-FDG) showed putaminal and cerebellar hypermetabolism associated with diffuse cortical hypometabolism. These findings were compatible with autoimmune encephalitis [64]. In a case series, four patients after 0–12 days from COVID-19 onset showed psychomotor agitation or slowing, accompanied by other signs, such as frontal lobe syndrome, cerebellar syndrome, status epilepticus, anxiety, and depressed mood. The PET/CT imaging demonstrated frontal hypometabolism and cerebellar hypermetabolism. Based on the supposed immune mechanism, the patients were treated with steroids and/or intravenous immunoglobulin with an improvement of the clinical picture [65]. In another case series on seven patients, with new-onset cognitive and behavioral frontal disorders with central focal neurological signs or seizures, brain ^{18}F-FDG-PET/CT was performed in the acute phase, 1 month, and 6 months later. In the acute phase, PET/CT showed a pattern of hypometabolism in a widespread cerebral network including the frontal cortex, anterior cingulate, insula, and caudate nucleus. At the 6-month follow-up, there was an overall clinical improvement, with variable residual cognitive and emotional disorders. CT/PET showed an improvement in brain metabolism with less cortical hypometabolism and no hypermetabolic areas. Overall, after 6 months, three patients showed a return to almost normal values, three other patients had a moderate improvement with persisting prefrontal hypometabolism, and one patient a severe hypometabolism in the bilateral occipital cortex associated with prefrontal and cerebellar hypermetabolism. Probably, a para-infectious cytokine release or cell-mediated immune mechanism involving the areas implicated in emotional and behavioral regulation, as well as cognition, fear, and anxiety-related regions, is involved. On these premises, in suspected encephalopathy, the use of PET/CT can offer a better correlation with clinical symptomatology monitoring than MRI [66].

3.2.10 Other Diagnostic Approaches

Although in many clinical conditions such as ischemic stroke, encephalitis, and hypoxic injury, CT and MRI studies are essential for correct diagnosis and effective treatment, other diagnostic tools can be easily and effectively used to monitor the clinical evolution, even in patients under sedation. Transcranial cerebral Doppler (TCD) could offer information on intracranial pressure or cerebral perfusion, near-infrared spectroscopy (NIRS) could provide information on cortical oxygenation, while automated pupillometry could aid to choose more carefully an adequate level of sedation [67]. Using TCD sonography and B-mode transcranial color-coded duplex (TCCD) could allow the evaluation of CBF velocity, cerebral autoregulation, critical closing pressure, and cerebral compliance, as well as the direct visualization of brain parenchyma, and cerebral arteries. Of interest in COVID-19 patients, a bedside evaluation of brain midline shift (MLS), optical nerve sheath diameter, arterial stenosis and recanalization, and vasospasm can aid the physician in the early detection and prompt treatment of such complications [68]. Non-invasive neuromonitoring through transcranial Doppler, optic nerve sheath diameter, and automated pupillometry can help to detect high intracranial pressure (ICP) in up to 40% of patients, and altered pupillary reactivity in 31% of the patients. These data confirm the importance of non-invasive monitoring in the early detection of severe complications [69].

In brief, data from the literature highlight that because of the high incidence and the wide range of neurological complications in COVID-19 patients, early use of neuroimaging studies is suggested. This approach is valid to better define the type and extent of nervous tissue damage. Furthermore, the clinical picture, supplemented by the neuroimaging findings and laboratory tests, could allow clinicians to identify the pathologic mechanisms and make a targeted treatment.

3.3 Electrodiagnostic Tests

3.3.1 EEG: Indications, Approaches, Features, and Limitations

Although EEG is commonly used for the evaluation of neurological patients, the increasing number of neuroimaging studies, mainly MRI, have reduced their indication to a more specific evaluation [70]. Furthermore, the pandemic has further reduced its use because of the increased risk of exposure to coronavirus of the neurophysiology technician during the long-term continuous EEG monitoring [71, 72]. Nevertheless, in the most severe cases of COVID-19, numerous neurological complications could benefit from timely and thorough EEG studies. These approaches can be useful to evaluate the clinical evolution and the response to therapy. Moreover, during the pandemic, the risk of undertreatment in known epileptic patients could generate a burden of psychological distress and lead to poor control of epileptic symptoms [73].

Thus, despite the abovementioned problems, the EEG study remains an indispensable tool in cases of altered mentation or seizure-like manifestations. It mostly concerns subtle conditions, such as the non-convulsive status epilepticus.

In COVID-19 critically ill patients, the most common indication is an altered level of consciousness (Fig. 3.5). In a case series, the EEGs acquired at bedside over 20–30 min showed a widespread slow activity (mainly delta) with a mild anterior emphasis, and sometimes, focal EEG abnormalities. These findings comprised intermittent irregular slow waves over both hemispheres with anterior emphasis, occasional anterior sharp waves, frequent triphasic waves with a leading sharp wave component, and irregular slow waves with anterior emphasis, peaked and triphasic. Probably, these EEG abnormalities can be ascribed to non-specific causes, such as hypoxia, sepsis, or metabolic derangement; on the other hand, focal disturbances can be related to some complications of SARS-CoV-2 infection, such as cerebrovascular or autoimmune insult, or co-existing pathologies [74].

Chen et al. [75] described five critically ill COVID-19 patients who underwent a rapid-EEG exam because of altered mentation and/or seizure-like manifestations. All patients showed some degree of diffuse slowing, and generalized rhythmic delta activity; two patients showed also generalized periodic discharge. These alterations consisted of bifrontal predominant continuous spike and slow-wave discharges up to 3 Hz associated with myoclonic movements in one patient, and generalized periodic discharges at 1 Hz and occasional burst at 2–3 Hz (resembling a non-convulsive status epilepticus), in the other one [75]. Other authors used quantified

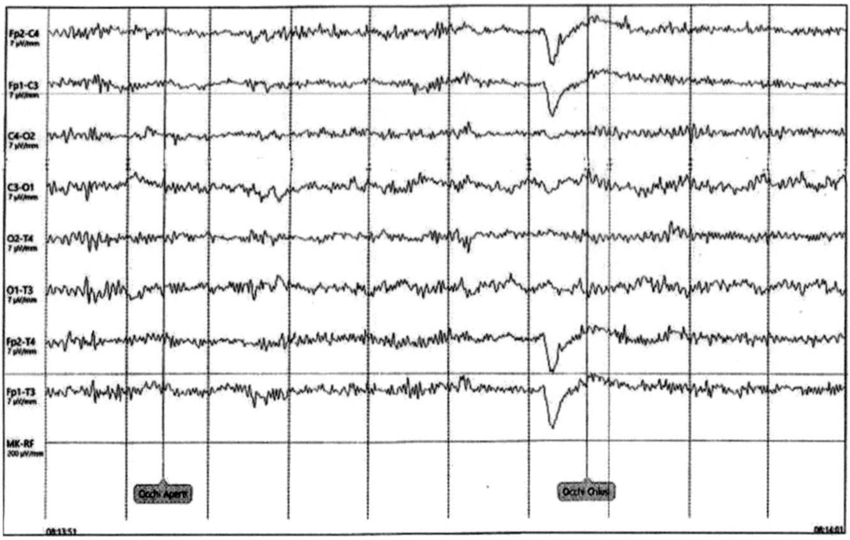

Fig. 3.5 Electroencephalographic examination in a 45-year-old man with an altered level of consciousness. The trace shows a basically low voltage background rhythm with widespread rapid rhythms and sporadic slow waves in the bilateral temporal region

electroencephalography (qEEG) to define specific patterns in COVID-19 patients after the release from the ICU. Twenty patients were analyzed and compared with two control groups of post-anoxic encephalopathy, and mild/moderate cognitive impairment. In COVID patients, they found a mean voltage and posterior dominant rhythm in the theta band; conversely, the EEG registered a tendency toward higher amplitude and slower posterior component in patients with cognitive impairment, and an amplitude similar to COVID and frequency comparable to cognitive impairment in post-anoxic encephalopathy patients. The mean frequency was statistically different in COVID, while the amplitude was similar in the three groups. Furthermore, compared to the patients with the cognitive impairment and post-anoxic encephalopathy, Shannon's spectral entropy (SSE), used to characterize the spectral complexity, showed higher relative amounts of faster bands (α and β) in COVID-19; again, the hemispheric connectivity was lower in COVID patients and there was a scarce presence of irritative activity. Although some common factors, such as hypoxia, could have a role in the EEG pattern of all three clinical conditions, it is reasonable to assume that some severe COVID patients could develop an encephalopathy with specific EEG features [76].

In another retrospective analysis, the most common indications of EEG were confusion and general, or focal seizures. In 21.8% of the patients, EEG was normal, in 21.4% it showed slight deceleration without spatial organization, in 19% non-specific abnormalities or questionable elements, in 9.5% focal or diffuse epileptic EEG (diffuse spike and polyspikes, frontal spikes, temporal, and rolandic slow sharp waves or spikes and wave spikes, and altered sharp waves), and in 21.4%

encephalopathic pattern (continuous or rhythmic frontal or diffuse slow diphasic or triphasic waves or sharp waves). Among the patients with confusion/psychomotor retardation, 85% of cases showed a modified pattern such as an encephalopathic-type pattern, or non-specific features. Moreover, among the patients with epileptic symptoms, in 57% of cases EEGs were altered (e.g., encephalopathic or epileptic patterns). In patients with brief loss of consciousness, only 20% had pathologic findings with slowdown or an encephalopathic pattern. The EEG of the two patients with hallucinations was normal in one patient and slowed, in the other one. The only patient with the suspect transitory ischemic cerebrovascular attack had a normal EEG. Taken together, a multifactorial pathophysiological mechanism is probably underlying these EEG findings. It may include direct viral involvement, and other factors such as cerebrovascular involvement, toxic encephalopathy, residual sedation, and the effect of hypoxia [77].

A multi-center prospective observational study evaluated the incidence and prognostic value of EEG findings in COVID-19 patients (60% in ICU). Indications were the unexplained loss of consciousness and/or suspicion of seizures. CT was performed in 67.7% and MRI in 25.8% of patients with neuroimaging injury present in 41.9% of patients (stroke, cerebral venous thrombosis, hematoma, SAH, edema, and PRES). Concordant lateralization of abnormalities between EEG and MRI was found in 29.8% of cases. The most frequent EEG finding was the generalized continuous slow wave delta activity (66%) followed by generalized intermittent slow waves (36.2%). In about 20% of cases, non-convulsive status epilepticus, seizures, and interictal epileptiform discharges were also observed. Periodic patterns were found in 3.2% of cases. Interestingly, the intercritical activity was generalized in 21% of cases, while the focal localization was more frequent in the frontal lobe (86%) followed by temporal (36%), parietal (21%), and occipital (21%) lobes. A multivariate analysis found that independent risk factors for mortality were cancer and the need for an EEG during the third week of the evolution of the disease. This last feature could be related to the occurrence of cytokine storm in this phase of the disease; it could lead to a deterioration of the clinical picture, and the onset of neurological symptomatology that, finally, is an expression of more severe disease with a worse prognosis [78].

Focal epileptic attacks were also reported. A 73-year-old man with mild respiratory symptoms and two episodes of painful muscle stiffening and twitching in the left arm and leg, lasting few seconds without loss of consciousness, was admitted to the hospital. During the stay, the respiratory symptomatology worsened and other episodes of similar cramp attack appeared. Brain CT and MRI showed a dilated ventricular system with prominent fissures and sulci and scattered white matter hypodensities. The CSF analysis highlighted slightly elevated leucocytes. The EEG was normal. After antiepileptic and symptomatic therapy, the clinical picture improved [79]. The first case of documented non-lesional status epilepticus was described in a 59-year-old patient who showed short episodes of impaired consciousness, confusion, and behavioral disturbances. The EEG demonstrated background fluctuating alertness with preserved responses to simple orders, and two widespread long rhythmic delta discharges, with superimposed spikes in predominantly frontal localization simultaneous with impaired awareness. The CSF and MRI were normal, and after the beginning of antiepileptic therapy, the follow-up EEG showed no alteration. Diagnosis of COVID-associated seizures without any underlying meningitis or encephalitis was made. This case underlines the importance of EEG study in COVID-19 patients with alteration of consciousness [80].

Other cases of de novo status epilepticus without a history of epilepsy were described. The use of a continuous video EEG in a patient with lethargy and disorientation demonstrated a severe background slowing, and multiple seizures emanating from the midline and left frontocentral regions, correlated with facial twitching, the head version to the right followed by a bilateral tonic-clonic seizure. Another patient featuring a reduced level of consciousness, and face and arm myoclonus, showed a marked background voltage attenuation and slowing, and continuous 0.5–0.75 Hz bilateral independent periodic discharges over the left and right hemisphere. The latter developed to form recurrent discrete seizures, emanating from either right or left frontocentral-parietal regions. Of note, both patients had significant comorbidities and unremarkable findings at neuroimaging. These cases offer further proof that in patients with fluctuating consciousness, the suspicion of subclinical status epilepticus should induce a thorough EEG study, even when mild respiratory symptomatology manifests [81]. The incidence and risk of acute symptomatic seizures were investigated in a multi-center retrospective study. The most frequent risk factor was hypoxia, followed by imipenem use, sepsis, shock, and multiorgan failure. None of the patients had a history of epilepsy, seizures, or status epilepticus during hospitalization. Only two patients had seizure-like events ascribed to acute stress reaction, in one, and hypocalcemia, in the other. The authors concluded that COVID-19 patients have a low risk to develop seizures, even in most critical cases. Nevertheless, clinicians should be aware of this critical condition, mainly in severe patients, to promptly minimize risk factors [82].

A retrospective study focused on the characteristics of EEG performed in COVID patients to find specific alterations. The most frequent indications were the absence of awakening after the suspension of sedation, confusion, or fluctuating consciousness, followed by suspicion of seizures, and other reasons. The authors evaluated 40 EEGs (collected over 20 min) from 36 patients (18 admitted in ICU) and described five classes:

- Normal findings.
- Class A (mildly altered): slow background activity within a theta frequency, preserved anteroposterior gradient and reactivity, without abnormal patterns.
- Class B (moderately altered): slow background activity within a theta frequency, preserved reactivity, and intrusion of sporadic, rare, or occasional slow waves of diphasic/triphasic aspect.
- Class C (severely altered): continuous slow background activity, preserved reactivity, and presence of abundant periodic or rhythmic patterns.
- Class D (critically altered): discontinuous background or continuous periodic/rhythmic patterns/continuous slow background activity with absent reactivity.

Epileptiform aspects, such as spike and waves, subclinical or focal seizures, or lateralized periodic discharges were not identified in all patients. Four EEGs were normal. Among the remaining 36 pathological EEGs, 52.7% were assigned to class A, 11.1% to class B, 22.2% to class C, and 13.8% to class D. In conclusion the majority of EEGs (57.7%) was found normal or mildly altered, mainly in patients admitted to the general ward, while 42.5% of EEGs showed more severe findings, mainly in ICU patients. The abnormalities were sporadic triphasic waves, multifocal or generalized periodic discharges, and rhythmic delta activity. The authors concluded it was not possible to identify a specific pattern [83].

Waters et al. [84] studied extensively the incidence of electrographic seizures and their risk factors. They discussed the potential indications for continuous EEG (cEEG) monitoring. They referred to generalized or focal acute hyperkinetic movements, altered mental status, reduced or fluctuating level of consciousness, and persistent coma after the discontinuation of sedative medications. In their series, the authors found seizures on EEG exam in 8%. In these patients, 30% manifested a non-convulsive status epilepticus. There was a history of seizure only in 8.9% of patients (50% of patients with a seizure on EEG vs. 5.5% of patients without seizure) and chronic brain disease in 30% (66.7% with a seizure on EEG vs. 27.4% of patients without seizure). The most common EEG findings were as follows:

- Diffuse slowing or attenuation, in 98% of patients (100% in patients with seizure on EEG, and 98.6% in patients with no seizure).
- Focal slowing (not including bitemporal slowing) in 13.9% (66.7% in patients with seizures on EEG, and 9.6% in patients with no seizures).
- Generalized periodic discharges with triphasic morphology, in13.9% of patients (0% in patients with seizures on EEG, and 15.1% in patients with no seizures).
- Sporadic interictal epileptiform discharges, in 7.6% (33.3% in patients with seizures on EEG, and 5.5% in patients with no seizures).
- Periodic/Rhythmic epileptiform discharges, in 6.3% (66.7% in patients with seizures on EEG, and 1.4% in patients with no seizures).
- Non-Convulsive Status Epilepticus, in 3.8% (50% of patients with seizures on EEG).
- Focal slowing with triphasic morphology, in 13.9% (66.7% in seizure on EEG, and 9.6% in no seizure on EEG).

These results suggest that seizures represent a small percentage of patients undergoing continuous EEG monitoring during SARS-CoV-2 infections. Considering the risks of infection for the staff and shortage of resources during the COVID-19 pandemic, clinical and EEGs should be preferred to cEEG monitoring. In particular, history of hyperkinetic movements, chronic and/or acute intracranial disease, history of epilepsy, and routine EEG exam showing focal slowing and epileptiform discharges, could be sufficient indications to a cEEG monitoring [84].

The utility of cEEG monitoring in COVID-19 patients was also investigated by Louis and coworkers [85]. The authors studied COVID-19 patients (n = 19) who underwent cEEG for at least 24 h (median duration 2 days, range 1–6 days) and

COVID-19 patients ($n = 3$) who underwent routine EEG for less than 1 h. The indications were an altered mental status in 77.3%, and the presence of seizure-like events, in 22.7%. Five patients had epileptiform abnormalities on cEEG, and periodic discharges were noted in one-third of patients. Although in absence of a history of epilepsy interictal epileptiform abnormalities are rare, the higher proportion of patients with asymptomatic EEG seizures seen in this study could suggest a wider use of cEEG monitoring to better understand and treat these clinical conditions. In another study, the authors evaluated the prevalence of seizure and other pathological findings on EEG of 100 COVID-19 patients (77% in ICU, 70% comatose. Twelve percent with a history of epilepsy, and 38% with a prior history of brain disorder). Excluding the patients following cardiac arrest, the most frequent findings were moderate generalized slowing (57%), and epileptogenic abnormalities (30%), such as epileptiform discharges, periodic discharges. Seizures were present in 7% of patients (4% non-convulsive seizures). At the multivariate analysis, that independent predictors of epileptiform findings were a history of epilepsy (OR = 5.4, 95% CI 1.4–21, $p = 0.15$) and definite/suspected seizure before EEG (OR = 4.8, 95% CI 1.7–13, $p = 0.002$). Thus, seizures are rare and the evaluation of predictive findings could aid to optimize the resources and reduce the risk of infection in EEG technicians [71].

Other interesting aspects of EEG evaluation have been explored. In a systematic review of 62 studies, Asadi-Pooya et al. [73] evaluated the occurrence of new seizures in COVID-19 patients, the EEG findings, and the consequences of the pandemic on patients with known epilepsy. The authors confirmed that the most common indications of EEG exams were alteration of mental status and the new onset of a seizure. Although it was not possible to identify a specific EEG pattern in COVID-19 patients, an EEG pattern showing continuous, slightly asymmetric, monomorphic, diphasic, delta slow waves with greater amplitude over both frontal areas, and with a periodic organization, was frequently described. In COVID-19 patients with known epilepsy, the authors found conflicting results about the incidence and the outcome, even though it seems that patients with preexisting neurological problems could have a worsening of their condition and a more severe form of the disease. Furthermore, many studies underlined the reduction of the quality of the care, an increase of anxiety and depression, and social isolation in people with epilepsy. However, the use of tools, such as telemedicine and electronic portal, could improve the access to care and improve the quality of life in these patients. Other studies confirmed that the most frequent indication to EEG exam can be encephalopathy or altered consciousness after the suspension of sedation, and seizure-like activity. The most common findings seem to be generalized or focal slowing, and epileptiform discharges. Some variables, such as the presence of comorbidities, different levels of sedation, effects of hypoxic, and metabolic complications, should be taken into account in the interpretations of these results. Furthermore, during the COVID-19 epidemic, concerns about the risks related to the contagiousness of the disease could reduce the number of EEGs and their montage and duration. Nevertheless, in presence of suspicion of non-convulsive status epilepticus, which can affect morbidity and mortality, the use of cEEG monitoring seems to be suggested [86].

The wide spectrum of EEG findings in COVID-19 patients has been addressed by Antony et al. [87]. The authors reviewed 84 selected retrospective studies on 617 patients, and 911 EEG findings. Also, the most common indications were altered mental status (61.7%), and seizure-like events (31.2%). The EEG type was routine EEG, in 71.4% of patients, and cEEG, in 28.6% of cases. The EEG was abnormal in 88%, and non-specific/unclear in 5% of cases. Again, neuroimaging was altered in 36.6% of patients. It was not possible to make a correlation between EEGs and MRI. While the timing of EEG studies from the onset of disease was variable, the main indication for the early studies was seizures and cardiac arrest, while for the later studies was an unexplained encephalopathy. In patients with positive EEG findings, abnormalities were detected through cEEG in 96.8% of patients, and by standard EEG, in 85% of cases. Among the three main findings, background abnormalities were the most common (72.3%), followed by periodic and rhythmic EEG patterns (15.1%), and epileptiform changes, and seizures/status epilepticus (12.5%). The authors performed a sub-analysis of these categories as follows:

- Background abnormalities:
  - diffuse slowing (68.6%)
  - focal slowing (17%)
  - absent posterior dominant rhythm (10.2%)
  - decreased reactivity (3.2%)
  - slow posterior dominant rhythm (2.3%)
  - discontinuous EEG/burst suppression (2.1%)
  - lateralized asymmetry (2.1%)
  - background attenuation/ suppression (1.3%)
- Periodic and rhythmic EEG patterns:
  - generalized (5.7%)
  - generalized rhythmic discharges (5.2%)
  - lateralized/multifocal (3.9%)
  - generalized periodic discharges with triphasic morphology (2.9%)
  - lateralized/ multifocal rhythmic discharges (2.6%)
  - stimulus-induced rhythmic, periodic, or ictal discharges (SIRPIDs) (1.1%)
  - unspecified localization (0.6%)
- Other epileptiform changes and seizures/status epilepticus:
  - focal epileptiform discharges (5.7%)
  - generalized epileptiform discharges (4.4%)
  - status epilepticus (3.6%)
  - multifocal epileptiform discharges (2.1%)
  - seizures (1.9%)
  - unspecified localization of epileptiform discharges (0.8%)

In brief, a specific EEG pattern of SARS-CoV-2 infection was not found. The authors showed that the most common EEG finding was diffuse background slowing, indicating a non-specific encephalopathy, suggested by other findings, such as generalized rhythmic delta activity, and generalized periodic discharges with triphasic morphology. Epileptiform changes were also found, suggesting underlying cortical irritability. In the follow-up EEG studies, 56.8% of patients showed an improvement. Finally, the findings of EEG abnormalities in the frontal lobes, such as focal slowing, periodic discharge, rhythmic delta activity, and status epilepticus, could support the hypothesis that the virus, once entered through the nasal mucosa, subsequently spreads to the orbitofrontal region, and could be a potential EEG marker of COVID-19 disease [87]. This hypothesis was otherwise explored. It was suggested that some findings, such as frontal periodic discharges, together with anosmia, the olfactory bulb abnormalities at brain imaging, and the hypometabolism within the orbitofrontal cortex on functional brain imaging, could support the hypothesis of viral spreading from the olfactory pathway to the other regions of the brain, especially the orbital prefrontal cortex [88].

A recent meta-analysis (12 studies and 308 patients) confirmed the results of previous studies, showing that abnormal background activity was the most common finding, and seizure/status epilepticus was infrequent. The pooled proportions of the various EEG findings were as follows:

- Abnormal background activity: 96.1%.
- Generalized slowing: 92.3%.
- Discontinuous/burst attenuation or suppression/suppression: 5.33%.
- Generalized periodic discharges: 16.5%.
- Lateralized periodic discharges: 0.19%.
- Generalized rhythmic delta activity: 13.4%.
- Lateralized rhythmic delta activity: 0.96%.
- Focal slowing: 8.65%.
- Epileptiform discharges: 20.3% (with a history of epilepsy or seizures: 59.5%; without a history of epilepsy or seizures: 22.4%).
- Seizures: 2.05%.
- Status epilepticus: 0.80%.

From these findings, the authors concluded that in COVID-19 patients the most common indication for EEG study was encephalopathy. There was a high proportion of abnormal background activity, while the focal abnormalities were nonspecific and related to complications of the disease, such as stroke or encephalitis, or to preexisting neurological diseases. In this meta-analysis, the low proportion of seizures and status epilepticus was confirmed although epileptiform discharges were higher in patients with a history of epilepsy [89].

3.3.2 ICU-Acquired Weakness in COVID-19 Patients

ICU-acquired weakness is a well-known cause of prolonged mechanical ventilation and hospital stay. It occurs in a wide number of cases and affects the quality of life of the patients after the discharge from the hospital. Emerging studies have shown its role in critically ill COVID-19 patients and have emphasized the importance of electrodiagnostic studies to confirm the diagnosis. Critical illness myopathy (CIM), critical illness polyneuropathy (CIP), or a combination of the two underlies the symptomatology with different pathophysiologic mechanisms.

Electrodiagnostic tests can help in the differential diagnosis and for establishing the more appropriate preventive measures and treatment. Nerve conduction studies in CIM show reduced amplitude of compound motor action potentials with a preserved sensory response, while electromyography shows polyphasic motor unit potentials, with or without fibrillations. In the case of CIP, nerve conduction studies demonstrate decreased amplitude or absence of sensory nerve action potentials, as well as signs of axonal damage without demyelination [90].

In cases of technical difficulties, for instance, because of the lack of patient cooperation or the presence of abundant edema, other methods have been proposed. They include the comparison of muscle action potentials generated by the direct stimulation of muscle and nerves, and the peroneal nerve test [90, 91].

About the clinic, Tankisi et al. [92] presented the first case of critical illness myopathy because of COVID-19 infection in a male ICU patient. He experienced a weaning failure after 11 days of mechanical ventilation with severe symmetrical proximal and distal weakness, muscle wasting, and absent deep tendon reflexes. On day 65 of hospitalization, electrodiagnostic studies were performed, confirming the diagnosis of CIM [92]. In the first case series on 12 critically ill COVID-19 patients with the suspicion of ICU-acquired weakness (ICUAW), the authors evaluated CIP, CIM, or both. Nerve motor and sensory conductions of the upper and lower limbs and concentric needle electromyography (EMG) of distal and proximal muscles were performed in all patients and skeletal muscle biopsy in three. In all but one patient, the studies showed signs of critical illness myopathy (63.6%) and critical illness neuropathy (36.4%). None showed both signs of myopathy and neuropathy. Muscle biopsies indicated necrotic and regenerative fibers without inflammatory infiltrates, in a case, and atrophic and regenerative fiber, in the other two. There was not a distinctive feature of SARS-CoV-2 infection in these electrodiagnostic tests [93]. On the same topic, Madia et al. [94] described six ICU patients who were submitted to electrophysiological study because of the evidence of acute flaccid quadriplegia with preserved ocular and tongue movements, minimal distal movements of the hands, and no sensory problems. Notably, in all the patients, results showed myopathic abnormalities with fibrillation potentials and rapid recruitment of small, polyphasic motor units in deltoid or biceps, quadriceps, and tibial anterior, reduced compound muscle action potential amplitude with markedly prolonged duration, normal sensory nerve action potential amplitudes, normal F wave, absence of demyelinating features, and normal repetitive motor nerve stimulation. In another case series, two patients were admitted to the neurorehabilitation unit after 4 and 7 weeks from the onset of COVID-19 and ICU admission. Both the patients presented flaccid proximal tetraparesis and limb-girdle muscle atrophy. Motor nerve conduction studies showed normal distal latencies and normal conduction velocities. Distal compound muscle action potential (CMAP) amplitudes were decreased, and their duration was prolonged in median and ulnar nerves, in both patients. Sensory conduction velocities and sensory nerve action potential amplitudes were normal. Needle EMG showed spontaneous activity (fibrillation potentials) in one patient, and a myopathic pattern with short-duration motor unit action potentials increased percentage of polyphasic potentials, and early recruitment at voluntary effort in proximal muscles, in both patients. Both the patients improved gradually, with a residual reduced proximal limb strength, and reduced endurance during physical activity [95].

From these premises, the importance of a correct approach to neuromuscular disorders should be emphasized. It should include a deepening individual and familiar history to exclude other causes of primary or secondary neuro-muscular disorders, as well as any genetic cause. It is also important to know the medicaments used, such as steroids, chloroquine, azithromycin, and linezolid that could have a role in the onset of symptomatology. Furthermore, the potential presence of myasthenic syndromes or Guillain-Barré syndrome (GBS) and its variants must be addressed [96]. GBS represents the most common cause of flaccid paralysis; the classic form is an acute inflammatory demyelinating polyneuropathy (AIDP) with ascending weakness, loss of tendon reflex, and sensory deficits. Two more subtypes are described in the literature: acute motor axonal neuropathy (AMAN), and acute motor, sensory axonal neuropathy (AMSAN). In COVID-19 patients with myasthenic signs and/or symptoms, a pattern of demyelinating polyradiculoneuropathy was found in 77.4% of cases, axonal damage was found in 14.5%, and a mixed pattern was reported in 8.1%. Because of electrophysiological findings, 81.8% of subjects fulfilled the criteria for AIDP, 12.7% for AMSAN, and 5.4% for AMAN subtypes [53]. In a case series of five patients with GBS due to SARS-CoV-2 infection, electrophysiological studies showed a low amplitude of the compound muscle action potentials, and in two patients prolonged motor distal latencies. EEM showed fibrillation potentials [50]. In a patient with the symptomatology of fatigue, dyspnea during effort, slight diplopia, and ptosis in one eye after some weeks from the onset of COVID-19 symptoms, the electrophysiological study showed a 15% decrement in the amplitude of compound muscle action potential registered in the right nasalis muscle while stimulating at low frequency the facial nerve. These findings supported the diagnosis of generalized myasthenia gravis [97].

3.3.3 Mixed CNS/PNS Pictures

In COVID-19 patients, physicians should be aware of potential mixed CNS and PNS disorders. Chaumont et al. [98] presented a case series of four patients that during the weaning phase from mechanical ventilation showed CNS symptoms, such as confusion, psychiatric disorders, and PNS symptoms, as weakness, tetraparesis, myoclonus, muscle atrophy. In one patient, MRI demonstrated signs of ischemic stroke, while EEG showed non-rhythmic slow waves. Three patients had electrophysiological features of acute motor demyelinating polyradiculoneuropathy of the four limbs with delayed distal latencies and F-waves, slowed conduction velocities, and conduction blocks. One patient showed lower motor neuron involvement with denervation of the four limbs, normal motor evoked potential amplitude in both the upper and lower limbs. Finally, two patients had an additional decrease of sensorimotor potential amplitude compatible with a critical illness neuropathy [98]. When mixed CNS/PNS pictures develop, the wide range of clinical and electrophysiological finding could be due to several pathologic mechanisms of nervous tissue involvement. They can include direct cytotoxic effects and immune-mediated mechanisms [99].

In conclusion, despite the risks related to the pandemic and organizational difficulties, electrodiagnostic studies are a valuable aid to define the clinical picture and to start the appropriate treatment, for example, in patients with non-convulsive status epilepticus and/or reduced level of consciousness. On the other hand, it is essential to identify patients who may benefit from these studies, to reduce the risk of transmission of the infections, and the burden of work during the pandemic.

3.4 Laboratory Tests

The potential viral entry into the CNS through the cranial and peripheral nerve, or by the hematogenous route, along with hypoxic-ischemic and/or metabolic injury, and immune mediated damage, has been postulated as a potential cause of neurologic acute and chronic symptomatology. The study of CSF, although represents an invasive procedure, is of paramount importance to clarify the COVID-19 pathogenetic mechanism and optimize the therapy. Furthermore, the study of some biomarkers of CNS injury in the plasma of COVID-19 patients, and its correlation with CSF findings, could further aid the knowledge of the pathophysiological cascade, allowing a more precise diagnosis, and a better guide to therapeutic interventions [100].

In this context, Edén et al. [101] investigated the CSF biomarkers in six patients with COVID-19 and neurologic symptoms. They focused on the presence of the virus and measuring the number of white blood cells (WBC) and other inflammatory markers, such as neopterin and β2-microglobulin. Furthermore, they analyzed the IgG index, a marker of intrathecal antibody responses, and the ratio of CSF albumin to blood concentration (albumin ratio), as a measure of BBB damage. Finally, these authors measured the levels of neurofilament light chain (NfL) which is a neuronal cytoplasmic protein highly expressed in large caliber myelinated axons. Since the CSF and blood levels of NfL increase proportionally to the degree of axonal damage in a variety of neurological disorders, the measurement of NfL, besides serving as a diagnostic and prognostic biomarker, also can represent a simple and effective tool for monitoring the disease's course. Notably, the SARS-CoV-2 RNA was found in the CSF of 3 patients. None of the patients had CSF pleocytosis (WBC ≤ 3 cells/μL), while both neopterin and β2-microglobulin concentrations were increased in all tested cases. NfL was elevated in 2 patients and the albumin ratio and IgG index were found normal. These unusual findings can be the result of high values of soluble inflammatory markers without pleocytosis, BBB damage, and intrathecal IgG synthesis. In other words, it can be the expression of a multifactorial mechanism of damage seen in different stages of the disease and mainly linked to the systemic effect of infection and immune activation, rather than a direct viral invasion. These findings were confirmed in another study in 30 patients who underwent lumbar puncture in different stages from the first diagnosis of COVID-19 (5.9 ± 9.8 days, median 1; range 0–35 days). In all the patients CSF PCR for SARS-CoV-2 f was negative. In the majority of cases, the CSF showed a normal or slight increase in WBC count. CSF albumin ratio was normal in most cases, although in seven cases (most in the critical phase), there was a disruption of BBB. Oligoclonal bands were negative in about half of tested cases [102].

Other researchers evaluated the correlation between neurological manifestations and CSF findings in 58 patients divided into four categories: headache, encephalopathy, inflammatory neurological diseases, and GBS. SARS-CoV-2 was detected in two cases (both with an increased ICP). None of the patients presented with CSF glucose levels less than 40 mg/dL, and no difference was observed between groups. Although one-third of patients showed high ICP, there was no correlation with a specific neurological picture. Pleocytosis, predominantly mononuclear cells, was observed in 17.2% of patients, mainly in inflammatory neurological diseases (64.3%), and encephalopathy (4.2%), while increased proteins were observed in 27.6% (mainly in GBS, 50%), inflammatory neurological diseases (35.7%), and encephalopathy (29.2%). No differences in CSF total Tau protein and NfL were found between groups. The patients with inflammatory neurological diseases showed a wide range of levels of NfL, with the higher values associated with increased ICP, and total proteins values. The latter were associated with pleocytosis. Increased CSF cell counts were also associated with higher NfL levels in patients with headaches and the group with encephalopathy. In this latter group, the increased CSF total protein levels were followed by higher levels of total Tau protein and NfL, in addition to cell counts. The local B-cell response was evaluated by oligoclonal bands (OCB): 81.6% of patients had no OCB in CSF and serum, 10.5% had identical OCB in CSF and serum, 7.9% had OCB only in the CSF. All the patients with GBS had no OCB in CSF and serum. Based on these results, two distinct profiles correlated to the clinical picture of encephalopathy and inflammatory nervous system disease were suggested:

- Elevated CSF total protein, and increased total Tau levels. It is an expression of damage of cortical nonmyelinated neurons, as a result of cardiovascular diseases or other factors, such as hypoxia and sepsis.
- Inflammatory syndromes as an expression of demyelinating injury. They include meningoencephalitis, ADEM, and myelitis, and can express various CSF findings, such as pleocytosis, a mild increase of proteins, and high levels of NfL.

These findings suggest that there is a great diversity of CSF profiles, even in patients with the same neurological condition. Nevertheless, it could be supposed that the viral infection triggers the response of systemic inflammatory response and the infiltration of immune cells into the CNS. Finally, it leads to neuronal injury, as documented by the values of Tau and NfL proteins [103].

An interesting study compared the immune parameters in CSF and blood of COVID-19 patients with neurologic symptomatology to evaluate the presence of a compartmentalized CNS immune response to infection. The results showed a divergent immunological response in the CNS compartment, characterized by an increase in CSF, but not in plasma, of interleukin (IL)-12 and IL-1b. These interleukins are related to innate and cell-mediated immunity. There were T-cells increased cellular activation, a significant enrichment of B cells, and a different anti-SARS-CoV-2 antibody profile between the CSF and plasma of the same patient. Furthermore, a subset of COVID-19 patients with neurologic symptoms had an elevated burden of autoreactive antibodies in their CSF, even in the absence of other CSF and MRI findings of inflammation. It was hypothesized a compartmentalized immune response involving the innate and adaptive arms of the immune system, even in absence of conventional CSF and MRI signs of neuroinflammation [104]. Another study evaluated the correlation between SARS-CoV-2 infection and the evidence of immune-mediated neurological symptomatology. In all the patients, PCR for SARS-CoV-2 on the CSF was negative. Pleocytosis was present in about 10% of patients who expressed anti-contactin-associated protein 2 (anti-Caspr2) antibody limbic encephalitis, and para-infectious meningo-polyradiculitis. The CSF/serum albumin was above the median level for age in about 50% of patients. Oligoclonal bands were found in 7/12 patients (6 with the same pattern in CSF and serum and 1 CSF-specific). Serum and CSF onconeural and anti-neuronal antibodies studies showed the presence of anti-Caspr2 antibodies in serum and in CSF, in one patient; serum antiGD1b IgG titer showed values >1/199 in three patients. Taken together, these patterns could be consistent with para-infectious encephalitis and polyradiculitis and, in some cases, SARS-CoV-2-induced secondary autoimmunity [105].

Two systematic reviews evaluated the evidence of specific CSF patterns, the differences between CNS and PNS findings, the prognosis, and possible therapeutic options. Tandon et al. [106] examined 67 articles and 113 patients. CSF RT-PCR for IgM and IgG antibodies were reported for 78 patients and were positive in 12 patients. Elevated cell counts (>5 cells/mL) were found in 43% of the fatal cases, 25.7% of severe cases, and 29.4% of non-severe cases. Moreover, increased cell counts were found in 43.2% of patients with CNS symptoms, and in 16.7%, of patients with PNS symptoms. Again, CSF protein level was elevated in 59.1% of the patients with CNS signs, and 77.8% of the patients with PNS problems. Furthermore, CSF protein level was elevated in 74.5% of patients with non-severe COVID-19, and 68.6% of those with a severe COVID-19 infection (100% of fatal cases). In five patients, CSF IL-6 was measured and was found elevated in two non-severe cases and three severe ones of CNS manifestation but in none of the PNS manifestations. The results highlight that in COVID-19 patients with neurological manifestations, the most common CSF finding was an elevated level of proteins with occasionally mild lymphocyte-predominant pleocytosis. Since an elevated protein level in CSF was detected in all degrees of severity of disease, this finding should not be used as a prognostic biomarker, but it should be considered by clinicians when deciding when to initiate immune therapy.

Another review of 242 papers and 430 patients evaluated the possibility that CNS and PNS symptomatology could be related to direct viral neuroinvasion [107]. In this analysis, 75% of the patients showed symptoms localized to CNS, and 25% to PNS. Of 238 patients with CNS symptoms tested for CSF SARS-CoV-2 PCR, 17 (7%) were positive and 3 (1%) indeterminate. Among 65 patients with PNS symptoms, none was positive or indeterminate. Patients without a positive CSF SARS-CoV-2 PCR ($n = 58$), were tested with CSF antibodies to SARS-CoV-2, resulting positive in 42 cases (72%). Furthermore, in 114 patients who did not have a positive CSF SARS-CoV-2 PCR or positive antibodies to SARS-CoV-2, CSF oligoclonal bands were tested, with positive results in 1.75%. It reflects intrathecal antibody synthesis. It must be emphasized that these last results should be evaluated with caution because antibodies could be transmitted to CSF via a damaged BBB or could be autoantibodies. In 45 patients who were not submitted to the abovementioned exams, CSF immunoglobulins were found in 16 patients (36%). Autoimmune antibodies in CSF were tested in 77 patients and 5% showed positive results. Furthermore, WBC count in CSF showed values >0 cells/μL, or WBC/RBC ratio > 1:1000 or pleocytosis, in 66% of cases. In 7% of cases, the values were 21–100 cells/μL, all with symptomatology localized to CNS. Values >100 cells/μL were found in 2% of patients. Other biomarkers, such as IL-6, IL-8, and β2 microglobulin were measured in CSF of 57 patients, showing increased levels in 79% of cases. It suggests inflammation, axonal injury, and gliosis. Furthermore, the elevation of these biomarkers in CSF but not in serum in some patients suggests a compartment-specific immune response although these findings could be related to other causes, such as hypoxic injury, and/or viral neuroinvasion. Based on these results, it can be concluded that the neurological symptomatology could be attributed to various factors, such as hypoxia, stroke, inflammation, and immune-mediate injury. On the contrary, the CSF direct or indirect evidence of the potential neuroinvasion of SARS-CoV-2 is scarce.

The increasing number of GBS and its variants poses the need for a deeper knowledge of the underlying pathological mechanisms in the COVID-19 population. In a systematic review on 73 patients and 59 CSF analyses, the albumin-cytological dissociation was found in 71.2% of the cases with a median CSF protein of 100.0 mg/dL. Mild pleocytosis, with a maximum cell count of 13/μL, was evident in 8.5% of cases, while CSF SARS-CoV-2 RNA was undetectable in all tested patients. The anti-gangliolipid antibodies (anti-GD1b and anti-GM1) were positive only in one patient with MFS and in one with classic sensorimotor GBS [53].

The study of CSF needs an invasive procedure that could represent an obstacle because of the burden of workload of medical staff and the increased risk of virus transmission, as well as side effects related to the procedure. Nevertheless, the possibility to measure and monitor blood biomarkers of CNS injury represents an interesting way to evaluate the impact of disease on CNS, and the effects of therapeutic measures. Kanberg et al. [108] tested two biomarkers of CNS injury in the plasma of COVID-19 patients. The patients were divided into three categories (i.e., mild, moderate, and severe COVID-19 disease) and were subjected to a measurement of plasmatic concentrations of two biomarkers of CNS injury: NfL and glial fibrillary acidic protein (GFAp). The latter is a marker of astrocytic activation/injury. Patients with severe COVID-19 had significantly higher plasma concentrations of GFAp ($p = 0.001$) and NfL ($p < 0.001$) than controls. GFAp was also increased in patients with moderate disease ($p = 0.03$). In brief, the author found that GFAp values were higher in moderate and severe cases, while increased concentrations of NfL were found later in the disease's evolution, and mainly in more severe patients [108].

Another study evaluated the presence of anti-neuronal and anti-glial autoantibodies in CSF and serum to explore the hypothesis of immune-mediated damage of CNS. SARS-CoV-2 PCR in CSF was negative in all patients but a high level of IgA and IgG SARS-CoV-2 antibodies were found in serum and CSF of one patient, and myelin antibodies in serum of two patients. Moreover, NfL levels were increased in CSF of all seven tested patients. Again, CSF indirect immunofluorescence showed strong IgG binding in most patients at the level of vessel endothelium, perinuclear antigens, astrocytic proteins, and neuropil of basal ganglia, hippocampus, or olfactory bulb. These findings seem to support the role of autoantibodies against brain regions responsible for neurological symptomatology, and could be a guide for targeted immunotherapy [109].

The routine laboratory findings could help to early identification of patients with CNS complications and their severity. In a retrospective analysis, the authors evaluated the differences in laboratory findings between patients with and without neurologic manifestations. The patients with CNS symptoms showed lower lymphocyte levels (median 1.0×10^9/L vs. 1.2×10^9/L, $p = 0.049$), platelet counts (median, 180×10^9/L vs. 227×10^9/L, $p = 0.005$, and higher blood urea nitrogen levels (4.5 mmol/L vs. 4.1 mmol/L, $p = 0.04$). These differences were more pronounced among the severe patients (lymphocyte count: 0.7×10^9/L vs. 0.9×10^9/L, $p = 0.007$; platelet count 169×10^9/L vs. 220×10^9/L, $p = 0.04$; blood urea nitrogen 5.0 mmol/L vs. 4.4 mmol/L, $p = 0.04$). On the contrary, there were no significant differences between the groups in non-severe patients. Furthermore, patients with and without PNS symptoms showed no differences, while patients with skeletal muscle injury demonstrated higher levels of creatine kinase ($p < 0.001$), regardless of their severity, and higher neutrophil counts, lower lymphocyte counts, higher levels of C-reactive protein, D-dimer, and liver and kidney abnormalities. It suggests an inflammatory and coagulation activation with multiorgan damage [110].

In conclusion, the wide range of CNS and PNS symptoms make the diagnosis often difficult. The study of CSF, together with imaging techniques, could offer great help. Although only in a few cases, SARS-CoV-2 has been detected in the CSF, the evaluation of protein and glucose levels, and pleocytosis, together with the measurement of markers of neuronal damage, cytokine, and antibodies can further clarify many aspects of neuro-COVID-19.

3.5 Neuropathological Findings

Even if autopsies are difficult to perform, especially during a pandemic because of the risk of contagion and reduced medical and technical resources, it is not superfluous to underline that the neuropathological examination of brain tissues can contribute to dissect the CNS mechanisms of SARS-CoV-2 toxicity, providing, in turn, useful indications for new and more specific treatments.

Case reports and case series have described a wide range of neuropathological findings, from white matter and axonal injury to massive hemorrhage. Sometimes, the SARS-CoV-2 virus was detected in the brain tissue. A series of 18 autopsies, showed in 14 patients atherosclerotic lesions at the gross inspection without acute stroke, herniation, or olfactory bulb damage. In all patients, microscopic examination showed acute hypoxic injury with loss of neurons in the cerebral cortex, hippocampus, and cerebellar Purkinje cell layer. No thrombi or vasculitis was found. Some foci of perivascular lymphocyte infiltration were detected in 2 brain specimens and focal leptomeningeal inflammation in 1 brain specimen. Again, no microscopic abnormalities were observed in the olfactory bulbs or tracts. There was no immunohistochemical evidence of the presence of viral particles in the cytoplasm of neuronal cells although the virus was detected at low levels by PCR in 5 patients. These results have been attributed to hypoxic damage, in absence of signs of encephalitis or other direct virus damage [111].

In a case series from Germany on 43 patients with SARS-CoV-2, the virus was detected in the brains of 53% of examined cases. Viral proteins were found in cranial nerves originating from the lower brainstem and in isolated cells of the brainstem. In 13 cases (30%), there were gross macroscopic abnormalities. Among these cases, six showed fresh ischemic damage in the territory of the anterior, posterior, and middle cerebral artery, while cerebral bleeding or small-vessel thromboses were not found. An amount of 53% of cases showed mild-to-moderate brain edema (a sign of agonal changes). In 86% of cases, a variable degree of astrogliosis in all assessed regions was assessed. Activation of microglia and infiltration by cytotoxic T lymphocytes, expression of neuroinflammation, was pronounced in the brainstem, and cerebellum with little involvement of the frontal lobe, while meningeal cytotoxic T lymphocyte infiltration was seen in 79% of cases. As the authors stated, the presence of SARS-CoV-2 was not associated with the severity of disease, and other factors, such as cytokine storm, neuroimmune stimulation, and systemic SARS-CoV-2 infection, could be at the basis of the clinical picture [112].

In another case series on COVID-19 non-survivors (n = 17), the pathological findings showed cerebral hemorrhage in 8 patients, focal ischemia in 3, edema/vascular congestion in 5, diffuse or focal spongiosis in 10. Moreover, there was no evidence of encephalitis, vasculitis, neuronal necrosis, or perivascular lymphocytic infiltration. In this series, viral RNA was found in 9 of 11 samples evaluated [113].

A systematic review of neuropathological findings in patients with COVID-19 found 14 articles and 146 patients (127 with pathological study) [114]. The most common symptoms were altered mental status (43.8%), and delirium (28.1%), followed by cerebrovascular events (6.3%), headache, nausea and vomiting, aphasia, and ageusia (3.1%). SARS-CoV-2 reactivity was positive only in 15.1% of brain sections. Most patients tested negative for SARS-CoV-2 on immunohistochemical stains. No pathological findings of PNS involvement were reported. Macroscopic findings showed absence of gross abnormalities in 10.3%, diffuse edema in 17.1% (uncal and tonsillar herniation in one patient), chronic infarcts in cortical and deep areas (basal ganglia and brainstem), and in watershed areas in 2.7% of cases. Intracranial bleeding was found in the cerebellum, in three cases. Diffuse microglial activation and reactive gliosis, more pronounced in the brainstem and the cerebellum, were documented in 35.6% of patients. Furthermore, histopathological examination of specimens demonstrated hypoxic changes in 28.1% of cases, localized to the hippocampus, para-hippocampus, cerebellar Purkinje cells, neocortex, brainstem nuclei, olfactory bulb, chiasma, neostriatum, and spinal cord, with evidence of leptomeningeal inflammation in 4.8% of cases. Signs of the inflammatory process were testified by the presence of cerebral venous neutrophilic infiltrates (1.4% of cases), perivascular lymphocytic infiltrate (34.2%), perivascular degeneration and calcification (3.4%), and variable degrees of neuronal cell loss and axonal degeneration/injury (6.8%). Other aspects were recent microscopic cortical infarcts (16.4%), acute microscopic/punctate hemorrhages (10.3%), small-vessel ectasia with perivascular edema, and microhemorrhages (6.8%), and endovascular microthrombi (6.8%).

Based on all these findings, some pathophysiological mechanisms could be hypothesized:

- The common finding of brain edema could be the effect of the direct virus invasion and the host-specific response, as supported by the presence of inflammatory cell infiltrates.
- The presence of blood extravasated could be explained by the tropism of SARS-CoV-2 to the endothelial cells, and the accumulation of inflammatory cells, leading to endothelial cell death.
- The symptomatology of meningoencephalitis could be an expression of focal or diffuse cortical, brainstem, or leptomeningeal inflammation, with localized perivascular, and interstitial infiltrates neuronal cell loss, and axonal degeneration. Also, in these cases, either the direct viral effect or the host inflammatory response could be responsible.
- Intravascular microthrombi and multiple infarcts could be related to a procoagulant state and endothelial dysfunction, with hemorrhagic evolution in some cases.
- Ischemic lesions found in watershed zones could be related to hypoperfusion determined by hemodynamic instability, while microvascular injury in the subcortical and deep white matter could be the expression of global hypoxic damage.

Another review of the literature described the findings of 81 brain autopsies. A wide range of pathological findings were found, from ischemic changes to intraparenchymal bleeding to microglial activation and perivascular T lymphocytes, and macrophage infiltration. In few cases, electron microscopy and PCR, but not immunohistochemical stains, showed positive results [115].

In summary neuropathological findings confirm the central role of macro and microvascular involvement—either ischemic or hemorrhagic—in the genesis of the clinical picture. Furthermore, the evidence of infiltrates of cells and microglial activation could be explained by the host inflammatory and immune response. Therefore, the macroscopic and microscopic studies of the brain of COVID-19 patients represent another powerful tool to understand the pathological mechanisms underlying the multiform clinical findings in COVID-19 patients with neurologic complications.

3.6 Conclusions

The wide range of neurologic complications highlighted during COVID-19 pandemic raised the need for a more accurate study of these patients by integrating various diagnostic techniques. It seems to be useful to achieve an early etiological diagnosis, and to immediately start the best medical treatment. Nevertheless, several issues must be addressed. For example, the pandemic has had repercussions on the organizational response to the patients' needs, either for the general population or hospitalized patients. Patients with known epilepsy could have difficult access to care as a result of hospitals restrictions or because afraid to get infected. In the case of in-hospital patients, some diagnostic procedures, such as neuroimaging techniques or electrophysiologic tests, could be a challenge due to the increased risk of virus transmission to other patients and staff. These drawbacks are particularly important for ICU patients that could experience sudden deterioration of clinical conditions and a precise diagnosis could be lifesaving.

Therefore, each hospital should follow guidelines regarding the safe practice diagnostic studies during the COVID-19 pandemic. They should be based on some specific points, such as the urgency of the exams and the assessment of benefit/risk ratio. Furthermore, any prevention procedure should be rigorously adopted, utilizing personal protective equipment, and general precautions, reducing to minimum the number of persons involved and the duration of the study, and using disposable equipment if possible. Lastly, during COVID-19 pandemic it could be useful to introduce some technological improvements, such as virtual platform or telemedicine to provide timely care reducing the risk of infection.

References

1. Koralnik IJ, Tyler KL. COVID-19: a global threat to the nervous system. Ann Neurol. 2020;88:1–11. https://doi.org/10.1002/ana.25807.
2. Montalvan V, Lee J, Bueso T, et al. Neurological manifestations of COVID-19 and other coronavirus infections: a systematic review. Clin Neurol Neurosurg. 2020;194:105921. https://doi.org/10.1016/j.clineuro.2020.105921.
3. Iadecola C, Anrather J, Kamel H. Effects of COVID-19 on the nervous system. Cell. 2020;183(1):16–27.e1. https://doi.org/10.1016/j.cell.2020.08.028.
4. Wang Z, Yang Y, Liang X, et al. COVID-19 associated ischemic stroke and hemorrhagic stroke: incidence, potential pathological mechanism, and management. Front Neurol. 2020;11:571996. https://doi.org/10.3389/fneur.2020.571996.
5. Nannoni S, de Groot R, Bell S, et al. Stroke in COVID-19: a systematic review and meta-analysis. Int J Stroke. 2021;16(2):137–49. https://doi.org/10.1177/1747493020972922.
6. Baldini T, Asioli GM, Romoli M, et al. Cerebral venous thrombosis and severe acute respiratory syndrome coronavirus-2 infection: a systematic review and meta-analysis. Eur J Neurol. 2021; https://doi.org/10.1111/ene.14727.

7. Patel P, Khandelwal P, Gupta G, et al. COVID-19 and cervical artery dissection—a causative association? J Stroke Cerebrovasc Dis. 2020;29(10):105047. https://doi.org/10.1016/j.jstrokecerebrovasdis.2020.105047.
8. Morassi M, Bigni B, Cobelli M, et al. Bilateral carotid artery dissection in a SARS-CoV-2 infected patient: causality or coincidence? J Neurol. 2020;267(10):2812–4. https://doi.org/10.1007/s00415-020-09984-0.
9. Förster M, Weyers V, Küry P, et al. Neurological manifestations of severe acute respiratory syndrome coronavirus 2-a controversy 'gone viral'. Brain Commun. 2020;2(2):fcaa149. https://doi.org/10.1093/braincomms/fcaa149.
10. Zubair AS, McAlpine LS, et al. Neuropathogenesis and neurologic manifestations of the coronaviruses in the age of coronavirus disease 2019 a review. JAMA Neurol. 2020;77(8):1018–27.
11. Berlit P, Bösel J, Gahn G, et al. Neurological manifestations of COVID-19"—guideline of the German society of neurology. Neurol Res Pract. 2020;2:51. https://doi.org/10.1186/s42466-020-00097-7.
12. Ahmad I, Rathore FA. Neurological manifestations and complications of COVID-19: a literature review. J Clin Neurosci. 2020;77:8–12. https://doi.org/10.1016/j.jocn.2020.05.017.
13. Garg RK, Paliwal VK, Gupta A. Encephalopathy in patients with COVID-19: a review. J Med Virol. 2021;93(1):206–22. https://doi.org/10.1002/jmv.26207. Epub 2020 Jul 11
14. Edlow BL, Boly M, Chou SHY. Common data elements for COVID-19 neuroimaging: a GCS-NeuroCOVID proposal. Neurocrit Care. 2021;34(2):365–70. https://doi.org/10.1007/s12028-021-01192-6.
15. Vogrig A, Giglia GL, Bna C, Morassie M. Stroke in patients with COVID-19: clinical and neuroimaging characteristics. Neurosci Lett. 2021;743:135564.
16. Jain R, Young M, Dogra S, et al. COVID-19 related neuroimaging findings: a signal of thromboembolic complications and strong prognostic marker of poor patient outcome. J Neurol Sci. 2020;414:116923. https://doi.org/10.1016/j.jns.2020.116923.
17. Oxley TJ, Mocco J, Majidi S, et al. Large-vessel as a presenting feature of Covid-19 in the young. N Engl J Med. 2020;382(20):e60. https://doi.org/10.1056/NEJMc2009787.
18. Cavalcanti DD, Raz E, Shapiro M, et al. Cerebral venous thrombosis associated with COVID-19. AJNR Am J Neuroradiol. 2020;41(8):1370–6. https://doi.org/10.3174/ajnr.A6644.
19. Dorigatti Soldatelli M, Faria do Amara L, Cordeiro Veiga V, et al (2020) Neurovascular and perfusion imaging findings in coronavirus disease 2019: case report and literature review. Neuroradiol J 33(5):368–73. https://doi.org/10.1177/1971400920941652.
20. Pons-Escoda A, Naval-Baudín P, Majós C, Camins A, Cardona P, Cos M, et al. Neurologic involvement in COVID-19: cause or coincidence? A neuroimaging perspective. AJNR Am J Neuroradiol. 2020;41(8):1365–9. https://doi.org/10.3174/ajnr.A6627.
21. Helms J, Kremer S, Merdji H, et al. Neurologic features in severe SARS-CoV-2 infection. N Engl J Med. 2020;4:382.
22. Keller E, Brandi G, Winklhofer S, et al. Large and small cerebral vessel involvement in severe COVID-19. Detailed clinical workup of a case series. Stroke. 2020;51:3719–22.
23. Hanafi R, Roger PA, Perin B, et al. COVID-19 neurologic complication with CNS Vasculitis-like pattern. AJNR Am J Neuroradiol. 2020;41(8):1384–7. https://doi.org/10.3174/ajnr.A6651.
24. Conklin J, Forsch M, Mukerji SS, et al. Susceptibility-weighted imaging reveals cerebral microvascular injury in severe COVID-19. J Neurol Sci. 2020;421:117308.
25. Kishfy L, Casasola M, Banankhah P, et al. Posterior reversible encephalopathy syndrome (PRES) as a neurological association in severe Covid19. J Neurol Sci. 2020;414:116943.
26. Wijeratne TC, Karimi L, et al. Case report: Posterior Reversible Leukoencephalopathy Syndrome (PRES) as a Biologically Predictable Neurological Association in Severe COVID-19. First Reported Case from Australia and Review of Internationally Published Cases. Front Neurol. 2021;11:600544. https://doi.org/10.3389/fneur.2020.600544.
27. Parauda SC, Gao V, Gewirtz AN, et al. Posterior reversible encephalopathy syndrome in patients with COVID-19. J Neurol Sci. 2020;416:117019. https://doi.org/10.1016/j.jns.2020.117019.

28. Anzalone N, Castellano A, Scotti R, et al. Multifocal laminar cortical brain lesions: a consistent MRI finding in neuro-COVID-19 patients. J Neurol. 2020;267(10):2806–9. https://doi.org/10.1007/s00415-020-09966-2.
29. Franceschi AM, Ahmed O, Giliberto L, et al. Hemorrhagic posterior reversible encephalopathy syndrome as a manifestation of COVID-19 infection. AJNR Am J Neuroradiol. 2020;41(7):1173–6. https://doi.org/10.3174/ajnr.A6595.
30. Dias DA, de Brito LA, Neves LO, et al. Hemorrhagic PRES: an unusual neurologic manifestation in two COVID-19 patients. Arq Neuropsiquiatr. 2020;78(11):739–40. https://doi.org/10.1590/0004-282X20200184.
31. Moriguchi T, Harii N, Goto J, et al. A first case of meningitis/ encephalitis associated with SARS-Coronavirus-2. Int J Infect Dis. 2020;94:55–8. https://doi.org/10.1016/j.ijid.2020.03.062.
32. Duong L, Xu P, Liu A. Meningoencephalitis without respiratory failure in a young female patient with COVID-19 infection in downtown Los Angeles, early April 2020. Brain Behav Immun. 2020;87:33. https://doi.org/10.1016/j.bbi.2020.04.024.
33. Bernard-Valneta R, Pizzarotti B, Anichini A, et al. Two patients with acute meningoencephalitis concomitant with SARS-CoV-2 infection. Eur J Neurol. 2020;27(9):e43–4. https://doi.org/10.1111/ene.14298.
34. Ye M, Ren Y, Lv T. Encephalitis as a clinical manifestation of COVID-19. Brain Behav Immun. 2020;88:945–6. https://doi.org/10.1016/j.bbi.2020.04.017.
35. Chaumont H, Etienned P, Rozec E. Acute meningoencephalitis in a patient with COVID-19. Rev Neurol (Paris). 2020;176(6):519–21. https://doi.org/10.1016/j.neurol.2020.04.014.
36. Meppiel E, Peiffer-Smadja N, Maury A, et al. Neurologic manifestations associated with COVID-19: a multicentre registry. Clin Microbiol Infect. S1198-743X(20)30698-4. 2021; https://doi.org/10.1016/j.cmi.2020.11.005.
37. Zanin L, Saraceno G, Panciani PP, et al. SARS-CoV-2 can induce brain and spine demyelinating lesions. Acta Neurochir. 2020;162:1491–4. https://doi.org/10.1007/s00701-020-04374-x.
38. Brun G, Hak JF, Coze S, et al. COVID-19-white matter and globus pallidum lesions: demyelination or small-vessel vasculitis? Neurol Neuroimmunol Neuroinflamm. 2020;7:e777. https://doi.org/10.1212/NXI.0000000000000777.
39. Parsons T, Banks S, Bae C, et al. COVID-19-associated acute disseminated encephalomyelitis (ADEM). J Neurol. 2020;267:2799–802. https://doi.org/10.1007/s00415-020-09951-9.
40. Varadan B, Shankar A, Rajakumar A, et al. Acute hemorrhagic leukoencephalitis in a COVID-19 patient—a case report with literature review. Neuroradiology. 2021;11:1–9. https://doi.org/10.1007/s00234-021-02667-1.
41. Poyiadji N, Shahin G, Noujaim D, Stone M, Patel S, Griffith B. COVID-19-associated acute hemorrhagic necrotizing encephalopathy: imaging features. Radiology. 2020;296(2):E119–20. https://doi.org/10.1148/radiol.2020201187.
42. Sawlania V, Scottonc,S, Nadera,K, et al (2021) COVID-19-related intracranial imaging findings: a large single-Centre experience. Clin Radiol 76, 108e116.
43. Munz M, Wessendorf S, Koretsis G, et al. Acute transverse myelitis after COVID-19 pneumonia. J Neurol. 2020;26:1–2.
44. AlKetbi R, AlNuaimi D, AlMulla M, et al. Acute myelitis as a neurological complication of Covid-19: a case report and MRI findings. Radiol Case Rep. 2020;15(9):1591–5.
45. Canavero I, Valentino F, Colombo E, et al. Acute myelopathies associated to SARS-CoV-2 infection: viral or immune-mediated damage? Travel Med Infect Dis. 2021;40:102000.
46. Ladopoulos T, Zand R, Shahjouei S, et al. COVID-19: neuroimaging features of a pandemic. J Neuroimaging. 2021:1–16. https://doi.org/10.1111/jon.12819.
47. Rodríguez de Antonio LA, Gonzalez-Suarez I, Fernandez-Barriuso I, et al. Para-infectious anti-GD2/GD3 IgM myelitis during the Covid-19 pandemic: case report and literature review. Mult Scler Relat Disord. 2021;49:102783.
48. Fernandez CE, Colin K, Franz CK, Ko JH, et al. Imaging review of peripheral nerve injuries in patients with COVID-19. Radiology. 2021;298(3):E117–30. https://doi.org/10.1148/radiol.2020203116.

49. Ramani SL, Samet J, Franz CK, et al. Musculoskeletal involvement of COVID-19: review of imaging. Skelet Radiol. 2021:1–11. https://doi.org/10.1007/s00256-021-03734-7.
50. Toscano G, Palmerini F, Ravaglia S, et al. Guillain-Barré syndrome associated with SARS-CoV-2. N Engl J Med. 2020;382(26):2574–6. https://doi.org/10.1056/NEJMc2009191.
51. Lantos JE, Strauss SB, Lin E. COVID-19–associated miller fisher syndrome: MRI findings. Am J Neuroradiol. 2020;41(7):1184–6.
52. Sriwastava S, Kataria S, Tandon M, et al. Guillain Barre syndrome and its variants as a manifestation of COVID-19: a systematic review of case reports and case series. J Neurol Sci. 2021;420:117263. https://doi.org/10.1016/j.jns.2020.117263.
53. Abu-Rumeileh S, Abdelhak A, Foschi M, et al. Guillain-Barré syndrome spectrum associated with COVID-19: an up-to-date systematic review of 73 cases. J Neurol. 2020:1–38. https://doi.org/10.1007/s00415-020-10124-x.
54. Mehan WA, Yoon BC, Lang M, Li MD, et al. Paraspinal myositis in patients with COVID-19 infection. AJNR Am J Neuroradiol. 2020;41(10):1949–52. https://doi.org/10.3174/ajnr.A6711.
55. Beydon M, Chevalier K, Al Tabaa O, et al. Myositis as a manifestation of SARS-CoV-2. Ann Rheum Dis. 2020; 2020-217573; https://doi.org/10.1136/annrheumdis-2020-217573.
56. Scullen T, Keen K, Mathkour M, et al. Coronavirus 2019 (COVID-19)-associated encephalopathies and cerebrovascular disease: the New Orleans experience. World Neurosurg. 2020;141:e437–46. https://doi.org/10.1016/j.wneu.2020.05.192.
57. Paterson RW, Brown RL, Benjamin L, et al. The emerging spectrum of COVID-19 neurology: clinical, radiological and laboratory findings. Brain. 2020;143:3104–20. https://doi.org/10.1093/brain/awaa240.
58. Kremer S, Lersy F, de Sèze J, et al. Brain MRI findings in severe COVID-19: a retrospective observational study. Radiology. 2020;297(2):E242–51. https://doi.org/10.1148/radiol.2020202222.
59. El Beltagi AH, Vattoth S, Abdelhady M, et al. Spectrum of neuroimaging findings in COVID-19. Br J Radiol. 2021;94(1117):20200812. https://doi.org/10.1259/bjr.20200812.
60. Chen B, Chen C, Zheng J, et al. Insights into neuroimaging findings of patients with coronavirus disease 2019 presenting with neurological manifestations. Front Neurol. 2020;11:593520. https://doi.org/10.3389/fneur.2020.593520.
61. Choi Y, Lee MK. Neuroimaging findings of brain MRI and CT in patients with COVID-19: a systematic review and meta-analysis. Eur J Radiol. 2020;133:109393. https://doi.org/10.1016/j.ejrad.2020.109393.
62. Franca RA, Ugga L, Guadagno E, et al. Neuroinvasive potential of SARS-CoV2 with neuroradiological and neuropathological findings: is the brain a target or a victim? APMIS. 2021;129(2):37–54. https://doi.org/10.1111/apm.13092.
63. Gulko E, Oleksk ML, Gomes W, et al. MRI brain findings in 126 patients with COVID-19: initial observations from a descriptive literature review. Am J Neuroradiol. 2020;41(12):2199–203.
64. Grimaldi S, Lagarde S, Harlé JR, et al. Autoimmune encephalitis concomitant with SARS-CoV-2 infection: insight from ^{18}F-FDG PET imaging and neuronal autoantibodies. J Nucl Med. 2020;61(12):1726–9. https://doi.org/10.2967/jnumed.120.249292.
65. Delorme C, Paccoud O, Kas A, et al. COVID-19-related encephalopathy: a case series with brain FDG-positron-emission tomography/computed tomography findings. Eur J Neurol. 2020;27(12):2651–7. https://doi.org/10.1111/ene.14478.
66. Kas A, Soret M, Pyatigoskaya N, et al. The cerebral network of COVID-19-related encephalopathy: a longitudinal voxel-based ^{18}F-FDG-PET study. J Nucl Med Mol Imaging. 2021:1–15. https://doi.org/10.1007/s00259-020-05178-y.
67. Peluso L, Minini A, Taccone FS. How to monitor the brain in COVID-19 patients? Intensive Crit Care Nurs. 2021;5:103011. https://doi.org/10.1016/j.iccn.2020.103011.
68. Robba C, Goffi A, Geeraerts T, et al. Brain ultrasonography: methodology, basic and advanced principles and clinical applications. A narrative review. Intensive Care Med. 2019;45(7):913–27. https://doi.org/10.1007/s00134-019-05610-4.

69. Battaglini D, Santori D, Chandraptham K, et al. Neurological complications and noninvasive multimodal Neuromonitoring in critically ill mechanically ventilated COVID-19 patients. Front Neurol. 2020;11:602114. https://doi.org/10.3389/fneur.2020.602114.
70. Young GB, Mantia J. Continuous EEG monitoring in the intensive care unit. Handb Clin Neurol. 2017;140:107–16.
71. Pellinen J, Carroll E, Friedman D, et al. Continuous EEG findings in patients with COVID-19 infection admitted to a New York academic hospital system. Epilepsia. 2020;00:1–9. https://doi.org/10.1111/epi.16667.
72. Sethi NK. EEG during the COVID-19 pandemic: what remains the same and what is different. Clin Neurophysiol. 2020;131:1462.
73. Asadi-Pooya AA, Simani L, Shahisavandi M, et al. COVID-19, de novo seizures, and epilepsy: a systematic review. Neurol Sci. 2021;42(2):415–31. https://doi.org/10.1007/s10072-020-04932-2.
74. Canham LJW, Staniaszek LE, Mortimer AM, et al. Electroencephalographic (EEG) features of encephalopathy in the setting of Covid-19: a case series. Clin Neurophysiol Pract. 2020;5:199–205.
75. Chen W, Toprani S, Werbaneth K, et al. Status epilepticus and other EEG findings in patients with COVID-19: a case series. Eur J Epilepsy. 2020;81:198–200.
76. Pastor J, Vega-Zelaya L, Martin Abad E. Specific EEG encephalopathy pattern in SARS-CoV-2 patients. J Clin Med. 2020;9(5):1545. https://doi.org/10.3390/jcm9051545.
77. Besnard S, Nardin C, Lyon E, et al. Electroencephalographic abnormalities in SARS-CoV-2 patients. Front Neurol. 2020;11:582794. https://doi.org/10.3389/fneur.2020.582794.
78. Skorin I, Carrillo R, Perez CP, et al. EEG findings and clinical prognostic factors associated with mortality in a prospective cohort of inpatients with COVID-19. Eur J Epilepsy. 2020;83:1–4.
79. Elgamasy S, Kamel MG, Ghozy S, et al. First case of focal epilepsy associated with SARS-coronavirus-2. J Med Virol. 2020;92(10):2238–42. https://doi.org/10.1002/jmv.26113.
80. Balloy G. Non-lesional status epilepticus in a patient with coronavirus disease 2019. Clin Neurophysiol. 2020;131:2059–61.
81. Somani S, Pati S, Gaston T, et al. De novo status epilepticus in patients with COVID-19. Ann Clin Transl Neurol. 2020;7(7):1240–4. https://doi.org/10.1002/acn3.51071.
82. Lu L, Xiong W, Liu D, et al. New onset acute symptomatic seizure and risk factors in coronavirus disease 2019: a retrospective multicenter study. Epilepsia. 2020;61:e49–53. https://doi.org/10.1111/epi.16524.
83. Petrescu AM, Taussig D, Bouilleret V. Electroencephalogram (EEG) in COVID-19: a systematic retrospective study. Neurophysiol Clin. 2020;50(3):155–65. https://doi.org/10.1016/j.neucli.2020.06.001.
84. Waters BL, Michalak AJ, Brigham D, et al. Incidence of electrographic seizures in patients with COVID-19. Front Neurol. 2021; https://doi.org/10.3389/fneur.2021.614719.
85. Louis S, Dhawan A, Newey C, et al. Continuous electroencephalography characteristics and acute symptomatic seizures in COVID-19 patients. Clin Neurophysiol. 2020;131:2651–6.
86. Roberto KT, Espiritu AI, Fernandez MLL, et al. Electroencephalographic findings in COVID-19 patients: a systematic review. Eur J Epilepsy. 2020;82:17–22.
87. Antony AR, Haneef Z. Systematic review of EEG findings in 617 patients diagnosed with COVID-19. Eur J Epilepsy. 2020;83:234–41.
88. Vellieux G, Sonneville R, Vledouts S, et al. COVID-19-associated neurological manifestations: an emerging electroencephalographic literature. Front Physiol. 2021;11:622466. https://doi.org/10.3389/fphys.2020.622466.
89. Kubota T, Gajeraa PK, Kuroda N. Meta-analysis of EEG findings in patients with COVID-19. Epilepsy Behav. 2021;115:107682. https://doi.org/10.1016/j.yebeh.2020.107682.
90. McClafferty B, Umera I, Fye G, et al. Approach to critical illness myopathy and polyneuropathy in the older SARS-CoV-2 patients. J Clin Neurosci. 2020;79:241–5.
91. Latronico N, Giovanni Nattino G, Guarneri B, et al. Validation of the peroneal nerve test to diagnose critical illness polyneuropathy and myopathy in the intensive care unit: the multi-

centre Italian CRIMYNE-2 diagnostic accuracy study. F1000Res. 2014;3:127. https://doi.org/10.12688/f1000research.3933.3.
92. Tankisi A, Harbo T, Markvardsen LK, et al. Critical illness myopathy as a consequence of Covid-19 infection. Clin Neurophysiol. 2020;131:1931–2.
93. Cabañes-Martínez L, Villadóniga M, González-Rodríguez L, et al. Neuromuscular involvement in COVID-19 critically ill patients. Clin Neurophysiol. 2020;13:2809–16.
94. Madia F, Merico B, Primiano G, et al. Acute myopathic quadriplegia in patients with COVID-19 in the intensive care unit. Neurology. 2020;95:492–4. https://doi.org/10.1212/WNL.0000000000010280.
95. Versace V, Sebastianelli L, Ferrazzoli D, et al. Case report: myopathy in critically ill COVID.19 patients: a consequence of hyperinflammation? Front Neurol. 2021;12:625144. https://doi.org/10.3389/fneur.2021.625144.
96. Finsterer J. Comprehensive work-up is warranted for patients with severe COVID-19 and muscle weakness including respiratory muscles. Clin Neurophysiol. 2021;132:692–3.
97. Scopelliti G, Osio M, Arquati M, et al. Respiratory dysfunction as first presentation of myasthenia gravis misdiagnosed as COVID-19. Neurol Sci. 2020;41:3419–21. https://doi.org/10.1007/s10072-020-04826-3.
98. Chaumont H, San-Galli A, Martino F, et al. Mixed central and peripheral nervous system disorders in severe SARS-CoV-2 infection. J Neurol. 2020;267:3121–7. https://doi.org/10.1007/s00415-020-09986-y.
99. Paliwal VK, Garg RK, Gupta A, et al. Neuromuscular presentations in patients with COVID-19. Neurol Sci. 2020;41(11):3039–56. https://doi.org/10.1007/s10072-020-04708-8.
100. DeKosky ST, Kochanek PM, Valadka AB, et al. Blood biomarkers for detection of brain injury in COVID-19 patients. J Neurotrauma. 2021;38:1–43.
101. Edén CA, Kanberg N, Gostner J, et al. CSF biomarkers in patients with COVID-19 and neurologic symptoms: a case series. Neurology. 2021;96(2):e294–300. https://doi.org/10.1212/WNL.0000000000010977.
102. Neumann B, Schmidbauer ML, Dimitriadis K, et al. Cerebrospinal fluid findings in COVID-19 patients with neurological symptoms. J Neurol Sci. 2020;418:117090. https://doi.org/10.1016/j.jns.2020.117090.
103. Espíndola OM, Brandão CO, Gomes YCP, et al. Cerebrospinal fluid findings in neurological diseases associated with COVID-19 and insights into mechanisms of disease development. Int J Infect Dis. 2021;102:155–62. https://doi.org/10.1016/j.ijid.2020.10.044.
104. Song E, Bartley MB, Chow RD, et al. Exploratory neuroimmune profiling identifies CNS-specific alterations in COVID-19 patients with neurological involvement. bioRxiv. 2020.09.11.293464. 2020; https://doi.org/10.1101/2020.09.11.293464.
105. Guilmot A, Maldonado Slootjes S, Sellimi A, et al. Immune-mediated neurological syndromes in SARS-CoV-2infected patients. J Neurol. 2021;268(3):751–7. https://doi.org/10.1007/s00415-020-10108-x.
106. Tandon M, Kataria S, Patel J, et al. A comprehensive systematic review of CSF analysis that defines neurological manifestations of COVID-19. Int J Infect Dis. 2021;104:390–7. https://doi.org/10.1016/j.ijid.2021.01.002.
107. Lewis A, Frontera JG, Placantonakis DG, et al. Cerebrospinal fluid in COVID-19: a systematic review of the literature. J Neurol Sci. 2021;421:117316. https://doi.org/10.1016/j.jns.2021.117316.
108. Kanberg N, Ashton NJ, Andersson LM, et al. Neurochemical evidence of astrocytic and neuronal injury commonly found in COVID-19. Neurology. 2020;95(12):e1754–9. https://doi.org/10.1212/WNL.0000000000010111.
109. Franke C, Ferse C, Kreye J, et al. High frequency of cerebrospinal fluid autoantibodies in COVID-19 patients with neurological symptoms. Brain Behav Immun. 2021;93:415–9. https://doi.org/10.1016/j.bbi.2020.12.022.
110. Mao L, Jin H, Wang M, et al. Neurologic manifestations of hospitalized patients with coronavirus disease 2019 in Wuhan, China. JAMA Neurol. 2020;77(6):683–90. https://doi.org/10.1001/jamaneurol.2020.1127.

111. Solomon IH, Normandin E, Bhattacharyya S, et al. Neuropathological features of Covid-19. N Engl J Med. 2020;383(10):989–92. https://doi.org/10.1056/NEJMc2019373.
112. Matschke J, Lütgehetmann M, Hagel C, et al. Neuropathology of patients with COVID-19 in Germany: a post-mortem case series. Lancet Neurol. 2020;19(11):919–29. https://doi.org/10.1016/S1474-4422(20)30308-2.
113. Remmelink M, De Mendonça R, D'Haene N, et al. Unspecific post-mortem findings despite multiorgan viral spread in COVID-19 patients. Crit Care. 2020;24(1):495. https://doi.org/10.1186/s13054-020-03218-5.
114. Pajo AT, Espiritu AI, Apor ADAO, et al. Neuropathologic findings of patients with COVID-19: a systematic review. Neurol Sci. 2021:1–12. https://doi.org/10.1007/s10072-021-05068-7.
115. Al-Sarraj S, Troakes C, Hanley B, et al. Invited review: the spectrum of neuropathology in COVID-19. Neuropathol Appl Neurobiol. 2021;47:3–16. https://doi.org/10.1111/nan.12667.

Neurological, Psychological, and Cognitive Manifestations of Long-COVID

4

4.1 Introduction

Given that the coronavirus pandemic has infected millions of patients, multiple long-term adverse effects on different systems and organs can be produced [1, 2]. The most common findings include respiratory symptoms (breathlessness and cough), cardiovascular symptoms (chest pain, palpitations), generalized symptoms (fatigue, fever, pain), gastrointestinal symptoms (abdominal pain, nausea, anorexia), musculoskeletal symptoms (joint and muscle pain), and dermatological, ear, nose and throat symptoms. Neurological and psychological manifestations including cognitive impairment, headache, sleep disturbances, peripheral neuropathy, dizziness, delirium, depression, and anxiety are included among the possible sequelae of the disease.

These physical and psychological post-acute symptoms constitute what is identified as a "Post-COVID" syndrome, otherwise known as "Long-COVID," or Post-Acute Sequelae of SARS-CoV-2 infection (PASC) and affects many individuals after the acute course of the disease. The term long-COVID should not be related only to most severe cases, but it can include also the consequences of mild disease with less serious symptoms, such as fatigue, headache, muscle and joint pain, and palpitations [3, 4]. Moreover, many COVID-19 survivors have reported a non-specific post-viral syndrome with chronic malaise, diffuse myalgia, anxious-depressive symptoms, and sleep disorders [5].

The importance of a precise long-COVID or post-COVID definition is fundamental to furnish to the patients a guide for a prompt referral to the health care system. Moreover, health care workers can receive a tool that can be useful for correct approach and support of the affected patients. Finally, it is also important for both preclinical and clinical research aims. This definition should consider the wide range of symptoms, the fluctuating and relapsing nature of the disease, and the uncertainties concerning the diagnosis of the acute disease and its duration [3, 6].

M. Cascella, E. De Blasio, *Features and Management of Acute and Chronic Neuro-Covid*, https://doi.org/10.1007/978-3-030-86705-8_4

A generic proposed definition of post-COVID is "people who have recovered from COVID-19 but still exhibit symptoms for far longer than would be expected" [7]. Another definition underlines the beginning of the acute phase, defining the post-COVID patient as "not recovering for several weeks or months following the start of symptoms that were suggestive of COVID, whether you were tested or not" [8]. Greenhalgh et al. [9] introduced a time limit, defining post-acute COVID-19 as a disease that extends beyond 3 weeks from the onset of first symptoms and chronic COVID-19 when it extends beyond 12 weeks.

The definition of post-acute COVID was addressed by some authors. Alwan et al. [3], for instance, underlined the importance of a retrospective diagnosis of COVID-19 and proposed five criteria for the definition of post-acute COVID:

1. PCR or antigen positive test for SARS-CoV-2.
2. Positive antibody test for SARS-CoV-2.
3. Loss of smell/taste in the acute phase in absence of other causes.
4. Symptoms consistent with the disease in a period and location with a high prevalence of COVID-19.
5. Presence of at least one symptom during the acute phase and close contact with a confirmed case of COVID-19 around the time of onset.

Other authors have empathized several variables including:

1. Typology of the patient: hospitalized, non-hospitalized, or asymptomatic.
2. Presence of intrinsic factors: age, gender, comorbidities.
3. Presence of extrinsic factors: duration of hospitalization, admission in an intensive care unit (ICU), prolonged bedding, adverse events derived from interventions.

Furthermore, they proposed a distinction between the long-COVID type from the persistent COVID one. The former is characterized by the delayed but progressive improvement of the symptomatology (from 12 to 24 weeks), whereas the persistent subtype shows protracted and less likely susceptible to healing symptoms (over 24 weeks) [4].

The National Institute for Health and Care Excellence (NICE), the Scottish Intercollegiate Guidelines Network (SIGN), and the Royal College of General Practitioners (RCGP) developed the guidelines for managing the long-term effects of COVID-19, distinguishing:

1. Acute COVID-19: signs and symptoms of COVID-19 for up to 4 weeks.
2. Ongoing symptomatic COVID-19: signs and symptoms of COVID-19 from 4 to 12 weeks.
3. Post-COVID-19 syndrome: signs and symptoms that develop during or after an infection consistent with COVID-19, continue for over 12 weeks and are not explained by an alternative diagnosis.
4. Long-COVID: signs and symptoms that continue or develop after acute COVID-19, including both ongoing symptomatic COVID-19 and post-COVID-19 syndrome.

The authors underlined that the term "post-COVID-19" reflects that the acute phase has ended and the patient has recovered, while the term "syndrome" reflects multisystem clusters of symptoms, often overlapping, which can fluctuate and change over time [1].

Pending a precise taxonomy, in this chapter we will use the terms long-COVID and post-COVID as synonyms to indicate all the clinical manifestations (signs or symptoms isolated, or associated with syndromes) that persist after the resolution of the acute phase of the disease.

4.2 The Long-COVID Phenomenon in Numbers

Although many studies reported that 50–70% of hospitalized and 25–50% of non-hospitalized patients exhibit several post-COVID symptoms [4–6], the actual incidence of long-COVID is quite difficult to establish. In fact, the reported incidence of long-COVID is variable based on the categories of patients included, the symptoms considered, and the time of evaluation. Many confounding factors have been identified. Notably, the lack of a widely accepted definition of long-COVID seems to be the major contributing factor to the variability of the results. Another factor could be the difficulty to distinguish patients with severe COVID-19, who have only partially recovered with sequelae of their disease, from individuals with mild severity disease or ongoing symptomatology. Furthermore, the general population could experience symptoms related to other intercurrent infections or the psychological burden of the pandemic.

Small studies reported persistence of symptoms after 2–6 weeks from the onset of disease in one-third of patients. A study from Switzerland on 669 patients showed that at least 32% of those reported at least one or more symptoms. Fatigue, dyspnea, and loss of taste or smell were the main persistent symptoms [10]. In another study on 274 symptomatic outpatients, cough and fatigue were still present at the time of the interview 14–21 days after the diagnosis of COVID, respectively, in 43% and 35% of the patients. In this outpatient population, older age and multiple chronic medical conditions were associated with prolonged illness [11]. A study from Italy assessed the patients ($n = 143$) after a mean of 60 days from the onset of the disease. The authors showed that, comparing the symptomatology during the acute and post-acute phases, 12.6% of patients was free of COVID-19-related symptom, 32% had 1 or 2, and 55% manifested 3 or more symptoms [12]. In a survey on 8193 respondents conducted in the United Kingdom by the Office of National Statistics (ONS), the prevalence of long-COVID was 21% at 5 weeks and 9.9% at 12 weeks, with a mean duration of symptoms following the infection of 39.5 days [13].

In the first survey in the United States (US) on 640 individuals (4.4% hospitalized) with symptoms lasting over 2 weeks, most participants experienced fluctuations both in the type (70%) and intensity (89%) of the symptoms. A large number of participants experienced symptoms for 5–7 weeks. The most common symptoms were slight fever, cough, shortness of breath, tightness of chest, fatigue varying in severity, brain fog, chills/sweat, mild body aches, mild headache, trouble sleeping, and loss of appetite. Brain fog and insomnia were more frequent than cough. Other neurological symptoms were seizures, dizziness, and balance problems. This symptomatology was milder in the first week than in the second and third weeks but was consistently reported for up to 8 weeks [14].

In another survey from Belgium and Netherlands on 2113 COVID-19 patients members of two Facebook groups, multiple symptoms were present 3 months after symptoms onset. It was showed a progressive reduction of the number of symptoms which concerned mainly the non-hospitalized patients compared to the hospitalized ones. Fatigue and dyspnea were the most common symptoms; moreover, only 0.7% of the patients were symptom-free 79 days after the infection, while 2% had an increase in the number of symptoms [15].

A large international survey (n = 3762) investigated on the prevalence of 205 symptoms in 10 organ systems and evaluated the trajectory of 66 symptoms traced over 7 months. In this cohort of patients, 64% experienced symptoms for at least 6 months, and the probability of duration beyond 8 months was 91%. The peak of the number of symptoms was at week 2 for the patients who recovered in less than 90 days, and at month 2 for those who recovered over 90 days. Three clusters of symptoms with different time courses were identified:

- Cluster 1 [mainly ears, throat, pulmonary, and systemic symptoms] with an early appearance and a peak in the first 2–3 weeks and a decreasing trend.
- Cluster 2 [mainly neuropsychiatric, pulmonary, and cardiovascular symptoms], with a slow increase, a peak between weeks 6 and 8, and a slow decrease or unchanging probability over time.
- Cluster 3 [most of the organs and systems, mainly neuropsychiatric, cardiovascular, dermatologic, and head, ears, throat, except for pulmonary], with a rapid increase in the first 2 weeks followed by a plateau or a slight increase or decreased.

These findings confirmed that long-COVID is a heterogeneous condition that affects multiple organs and systems, and with a great impact on the quality of life (QoL) of the patients [16].

In addition to the clinical aspects, patients are worried and ask us for information on the duration of the manifestations of long-COVID. Although certainties will come from epidemiological and follow-up studies, some data on prognosis are already available. In a study on the general population in the US, a questionnaire was administered to 21,359 subjects with a history of SARS-CoV-2 infection. The results showed that about 36% continued to have at least one symptom after 30 days of the diagnosis, compared to 11.7% among those with negative test and 8.4% among those with no test. There was a further reduction at 60 and 90 days, respectively, to 25.3% and 14.8% for COVID-19 positive cases, 8.5% and 7% for COVID-19 negative controls, and 6.3% and 4.8% for those with no tests. At 90 days, COVID-19 positive cases were associated with anosmia, ageusia, chest, and joint/bone pain, and muscle weakness. Interestingly, dyspnea was associated with long-lasting symptomatology [17]. Furthermore, in non-hospitalized patients, Hellmuth et al. [18] showed that neurocognitive symptoms can be present for at least a median of 98 days after recovering from COVID.

Many studies highlight the long-term effects of COVID-19 on QoL and underline the need for programs aimed at supporting the full recovery after the hospitalization. In the study of Carfì et al. [12], a declined QoL at 60 days from the onset of the disease was found in 44.1% of the patients. In another investigation, 35% of respondents reported they had not yet returned to their usual state of health at the time of the interview [11]. An observational cohort study in 38 US hospitals evaluated clinical, financial, and mental health outcomes at 60 days post-discharge. Of 1250 patients, 78% were at home and 12.6% were discharged to a rehabilitation unit. At 60 days, 84 patients (6.7% of the discharged patients) died and 189 (15.1%) were re-hospitalized. Moreover, 11.8% reported difficulty in completing activities of daily living, 60% were able to return to work, with one of four reporting reduced hours or modified duties. Furthermore, 36.6% complained of a financial impact [19]. Another study showed a worsened QoL in 29.9% of patients, mainly in the inpatient group (43.8%), and less in the outpatient one (29.3%). Interestingly, also 18.2% of asymptomatic individuals complained an impaired QoL [20]. Other investigations reported that approximately 86% of respondents were mild to severely unable to work. In this cohort only about a quarter of non-recovered respondents and less than half (49.3%) of recovered respondents were able to engage the same number of working hours as before the illness [16]. Finally, Goërtz et al. [15] demonstrated that, compared to before the infection, the health status at the follow-up was significantly impaired. Age, previous health status, and the number of symptoms during the infection significantly predicted the number of symptoms at the follow-up.

4.3 Neurological Symptoms

4.3.1 Mechanisms

Understanding the precise mechanisms of post-COVID symptoms represents the first issue to be addressed. It could be difficult to distinguish the various causes of this multiform and often non-specific symptomatology. For instance, fatigue and dyspnea could be ascribed to direct muscle or peripheral nerve damage or be a result of the reduced cardiovascular reserve [1, 2]. Concerning neurological sequelae, multiple mechanisms, such as endotheliitis, cytokine storm, direct viral damage, and microthrombosis, can be involved [21, 22]. It has been postulated that the clinical picture of chronic-neuro-COVID could be linked to an ongoing low-grade inflammatory response and/or degeneration of functional neuronal and glial cells, while the vascular occlusion seems involved in the acute phase of the disease [23]. Interestingly, a study comparing the serum of patients 40–45 days after the infection to that of healthcare workers without infection, demonstrated persistence of the inflammatory response and mitochondrial stress [24]. Another small-size study (n = 24) evaluated the levels of cytokine and antibodies and neuronal-enriched extracellular vesicles (nEVs) after 1–3 months from SARS-CoV-2 infection The results demonstrated an increase of plasma interleukin (IL)-4 in all subjects, a positive correlation of IL-6 with age, severity of the sequelae, and increased values of SARS-CoV-2 antibodies. Furthermore, the protein markers of neuronal dysfunction were increased in the nEVs of all patients. These findings are suggestive of ongoing neuroinflammation with occult neural damage [25]. Finally, the so-called immunosenescence, found in frail elderly patients and characterized by chronic inflammation with an altered innate and adaptive response as well as endothelial dysfunction, could play a role in the persistence, or the new-onset occurrence, of neurological symptoms [5, 26].

4.3.2 Clinical Features

Neurological manifestations of neuro-COVID are manifold. Some of these symptoms and clinical manifestations, such as stroke, occur subacutely in the immediate aftermath of the disease. They represent a tail of the acute phase. Other conditions, such as fatigue, have a progressive course and are more properly labeled as chronic forms of PASC (Table 4.1).

Fatigue is one of the most common symptoms reported in the post-COVID-19. Its extent and duration remind the aspects of the chronic fatigue syndrome that was described after other infections such as the severe acute respiratory syndrome (SARS) and the Middle East respiratory syndrome (MERS) [8]. Rudroff et al. [27] defined fatigue as the decrease in physical and/or mental performance that results from changes in central, psychological, and/or peripheral factors due to the COVID-19 disease. Central factors include neurotransmitters level, intrinsic neuronal excitability, inflammation, and demyelination. Stress, anxiety, depression, and fear are psychological factors that could contribute to the occurrence of fatigue. Some peripheral factors such as pain and skeletal muscle weakness could be other important factors leading to fatigue.

In a survey involving 287 recovered COVID-19 patients, only 10.8% of all cases had no manifestations after the recovery, with fatigue present in most of the subjects (72.8%). The fatigue was followed by anxiety (38%) and joints pain (31.4%) while continuous headache, chest pain, dementia, depression, and dyspnea occurred in 28% of the participants [28]. In another study, fatigue or muscle weakness was found in 63% of patients after 60 days from the onset of acute symptomatology [19]. Similar results were also found during the hospital stay and at a 60-day follow-up. In particular, fatigue was the most reported symptom (53% of patients) either in the acute phase or during the re-evaluation [12]. In a study on 292 outpatients with mild COVID-19 disease conducted at 14–21 days after the test date by telephonic interview, 34% of those reported the persistence of fatigue [11].

These findings were confirmed even in a longer period of follow-up. A cohort study from Wuhan, China on 1733 discharged patients showed that 76% of patients reported at least one symptom at a 6-month follow-up. The most common symptoms were fatigue or muscle weakness (63%), followed by sleep difficulty (26%), anxiety and depression (23%). Female gender and older age were associated with higher levels of fatigue and muscle weakness, while the female gender and severity

Table 4.1 Neurological manifestations of long-COVID-19

Clinical manifestation[a] [Ref.]	Features	Occurrence[b]	Pathogenesis
Fatigue and muscle weakness [11, 19, 27–30]	Decrease in physical and/or mental performance that results from changes in central, psychological, and/or peripheral factors It may persist after 6 months	34–72%	Direct muscle or peripheral nerve damage or reduced cardiovascular reserve (oxidative damage)
Seizures [37, 38]	Focal motor, tonic-clonic, convulsive status epilepticus, and non-convulsive status epilepticus	2.8% (in those with neurologic manifestations)	Neuroinflammation (upregulated cytokines within the CNS)
Headache [13, 33, 34]	It is usually diffuse, pulsating or pressing, with moderate intensity, often accompanied by anosmia/ageusia, neck stiffness, nausea, and photophobia. Long-lasting duration and analgesic resistance	10–70%	Neuroinflammation, stressful conditions
Smell and taste disorders [11, 12, 29]	Hypo/anosmia, parosmia, olfactory hallucinations, fluctuating hyposmia dysgeusia/ageusia	11–20%	Damage of the cells of the olfactory epithelium or other sites of the olfactory system due to direct viral action or cytokine storm
Guillain-Barré syndrome [36]	Occurs 11–50 days from the first symptoms of the COVID-19. Ascending flaccid paralysis with areflexia/hyporeflexia, and sensory deficits	Case reports	Post-infectious immune response
Post-COVID stroke [1, 35]	Occurs days to 1 or more months from the first symptoms of the COVID 19	Case reports	Systemic inflammation and hypercoagulable state
Chronic pain [8, 15, 16]	Headache, muscle/joint pain, chest and abdominal pain, neuropathic pain. Worsening of preexisting chronic pain	34–44%	Multifactorial: Proinflammatory cytokines, direct/indirect viral damage

[a]Other neurological manifestations of post-COVID are sensorimotor symptoms such as tremors, numbness, facial paralysis

[b]Occurrence varies among studies occurrence varies according to the follow-up period considered (usually 60-day)

of illness were linked to persistent psychological symptoms. The authors underlined the need for longer follow-up studies and proper post-discharge care, at least in the more severe clinical presentations [29]. A study conducted on outpatients with mild or severe illness showed similar results. Fatigue was reported in over 60% of patients during the acute phase, either in mild and severely ill patients. Furthermore, fatigue was the most common symptom reported in the post-discharge phase (13.6% of patients) [30]. About the lasting of the symptom, Davis et al. [16] reported that its occurrence increases over the first 2 months of illness before plateauing and persists after 6 months. It was reported as the most debilitating symptom. On the other hand, the UK Office of National Statistics survey showed that among 8193 respondents the estimated prevalence of fatigue was 11.5 (95% CI 10.7–2.4) [13].

Other frequent non-specific symptoms include smell and taste disorders, diffuse muscle and joint pain, and headache. These symptoms are often combined with others such as fatigue and breathlessness [8]. After a 60-day follow-up, smell disorders were observed in 11% of the post-COVID individuals, taste disorders in 7%, dizziness in 6%, myalgia in 2%, and headache in 2% of those [29]. In another survey, joint pain was found in 31.4% of participants, continuous headache in 28.9%, blurred vision in 17.1%, tinnitus in 16.7%, and migraine in 2.8% [28]. Moreover, joint pain was the third and anosmia the sixth most reported symptom in the post-acute phase, while dysgeusia, headache, and myalgia were less reported [12]. In an international survey (n = 3762), the mean prevalence of smell and taste disorders was 57.6% and the prevalence of sensorimotor symptoms such as tremors, numbness, facial paralysis, weakness was 80.5% (95% CI 79.3%–81.8%) [16].

The incidence of each symptom varies among studies. The setting considered plays an important role. For example, the loss of sense of taste or smell was present in more than 50% of patients with mild illness and over 30% in those with severe illness during the acute phase. On the contrary, these percentages were reduced to less than 20% in both groups during the post-COVID period. Similarly, muscle or body pain was present in about 70% in both the categories in the acute phase and in less than 10% after resolution of the acute phase [20]. A study from the US on 292 outpatients with mild disease interviewed 14–21 days after the test date reported that the loss of smell and taste was present in more than 20%, and persistent headache and diffuse body aches in about 10% [11].

COVID-19 patients are at increased risk of chronic pain [30]. Dissecting the pathogenic aspects of this phenomenon is very difficult. Clauw et al. [31] have described three possible factors including the effects of post-viral syndrome or viral-associated organ damage, the worsening of preexisting chronic pain due to problems of public health response or personal issues, and chronic pain newly triggered in non-COVID patients submitted to risk factors, such as poor sleep, anxiety, or depression. Furthermore, Kemp et al. [32] have identified the following risk factors:

- *Population involved*: presence of comorbidities, older population.
- *Neurological insult*: neurotropism, immune response, painful neurological sequelae (e.g., stroke).

- *Mental health burden*: post-traumatic stress disorder (PTSD), social isolation, psychological burden of the pandemic.
- *Pain during the acute phase*: painful symptoms, procedural pain, low priority for its management.
- *ICU admission*: prolonged immobility, repeated prone positioning, neuromuscular block, procedural pain.
- *Rehabilitation issues*: overburdened rehabilitation services, organizational difficulties.

Probably, some SARS-CoV-2 pandemic-specific issues could increase the risk of chronic pain. For example, virus neurotropism and the psychological impact of isolation measures could play a central role in the pathogenesis of some symptoms, such as headache. Other risk factors such as prolonged immobilization, and procedural pain during ICU stay, could foster chronic myalgia, and joint pain [28, 32].

Combined with fever, cough, myalgia/fatigue, and dyspnea, headache is one of the most common symptoms of the acute phase; nevertheless, it can occur later, between the seventh and tenth days from the onset of symptomatology. Headache is usually diffuse, pulsating or pressing, with moderate intensity, often accompanied by anosmia/agcusia, neck stiffness, nausea, and photophobia. The duration is more than 48–72 hrs and, in the majority of cases, there is no or partial response to analgesics [33, 34]. Its prevalence was found up to 76%, with the most common manifestations being ocular, diffuse, and temporal. Almost a quarter of the patients reported headaches after mental exertion, while another quarter experienced migraines; among the latter, one-half did not suffer before [16]. About possible mechanisms, the viral invasion of the central nervous system (CNS) through nerve endings, and the effects of cytokine storm were postulated [33, 34]. In the ONS survey, headache was the third most common symptom of long-COVID after fatigue and cough, with an estimated prevalence of 10.1% (95% CI 9.3–10.9%) [13].

In post-COVID-19 patients chest pain is frequently reported, and requires a differential diagnosis between that of musculoskeletal and cardiac origin [8]. The prevalence of musculoskeletal disorders including chest tightness, joint pain, and muscle aches was 93.85% (95% CI 93.03%–94.60%) [16]. In another study in which chest tightness was investigated alone, a prevalence of 44% was reported [15].

According to the NICE classification, other clinical manifestations should be addressed among the sequelae of COVID-19 [1]. Stroke is another frequent complication either in the acute and subacute phases of the disease. Some authors have underlined the increased risk of cerebrovascular events in these patients. They recognized these complications as one of the most frequent causes of indirect CNS lesions [35]. Probably, post-COVID stroke is caused by systemic inflammation and hypercoagulability. Typical finding in patients with COVID-19 and coagulopathy is increased D-dimer concentration, a relatively modest decrease in platelet count, and a prolongation of the prothrombin time.

Other less frequent post-COVID manifestations were reported in the literature. Guillain-Barré syndrome (GBS) was described as a neurologic manifestation of SARS-CoV-2 infection, typically with an onset time ranging between 11 and

14 days from the first symptoms of the COVID-19. An interesting report described a case of GBS with an interval of 53 days from a COVID-19 pneumonitis. The patient, a 56-year-old man, was admitted for lethargy, sensory loss, distal lower-limb weakness, paresthesia, and severe bilateral leg pain. The cerebrospinal fluid (CSF) study showed a raise in total proteins, whereas brain and spine MRI were unremarkable. The clinical picture showed a progressive deterioration, with ascending weakness and breathing difficulties. The patient was admitted to the ICU and treated with non-invasive ventilation and intravenous immunoglobulin. He recovered gradually and was discharged home. The authors suggested that this long-time-interval supported the pathophysiologic hypothesis of a post-infectious immune response, rather than a para-infectious manifestation [36].

Finally, new onset of a focal or generalized seizure and status epilepticus were reported in the literature. In a large database on 40,469 COVID-19 patients, seizures were reported in 2.8% of patients with neurologic manifestations [37]. A recent case report described a 71-year-old SARS-CoV-2 man admitted for disconjugate gaze, ptosis, vertical diplopia, nausea, and vomiting. CT angiography showed a severe right vertebral artery stenosis with normal perfusion. The symptomatology resolved after thrombolysis and the patient was discharged home without neurologic deficits. Six days later, the patient returned to the hospital confused and incontinent. A brain CT showed new hyperemia in the bilateral frontal lobes. Brain MRI, CSF, and blood test were unremarkable, while a new PCR test for SARS-CoV-2 was negative. The suspect of seizures was confirmed by the electroencephalography that demonstrated several seizure manifestations. These seizures were lateralized, right central predominant, and sharply contoured rhythmic delta activity at 1–3 Hz that spread to the temporal, then frontal lobes bilaterally. The patient was treated with anti-epileptics and discharged home. Probably, these findings were related to a lingering inflammation and upregulated cytokines within the CNS [38].

Practical Therapeutic Suggestions for Addressing Chronic COVID-Pain

Currently, there is no cure for long-term COVID. Tailored multimodal through the combination of pharmacological and non-pharmacological strategies:

- Acetaminophen or NSAIDs (for short periods and not contraindicated).
- Opioids (unless in patients who already use these drugs for chronic pain) must be avoided.
- Patients who depend on chronic steroids should not have the medication discontinued. Moreover, at resolution of the acute phase of COVID, steroids for the management of diffuse musculoskeletal pain (through short-duration cycles) can be used.
- Muscle relaxants (e.g., cyclobenzaprine) can help muscle spasm.
- Antidepressant medications (e.g., amitriptyline, duloxetine, venlafaxine, fluoxetine).
- Anticonvulsants (e.g., low dose gabapentinoids) for painful neuropathies.

- Vitamin B and neurotropic (e.g., palmitoylethanolamide) .
- Non-pharmacological strategies (e.g., acupuncture, physical therapy, psychological support, relaxation techniques).

In particular, tailored therapies with dynamic multimodal approaches must follow:

- Pain features.
- Its potential physiopathology.
- The complexity of the symptoms.
- The impact on the health-related quality of life.
- Comorbidities.
- Psychological aspects and social context.

4.4 Psychological Sequelae of Long-COVID

4.4.1 Disease-Related or Pandemic-Induced Effects?

The emergency caused by COVID-19 has impacted every aspect of life, including work, school, and sociality. Thus, the pandemic is a relevant psychological stressor. It can induce very important psychological effects even in those who have not been infected with the virus. Physical distancing measures such as self-isolation or quarantine are, probably, the main causes of stress. In this regard, it has been estimated that about 4 in 10 adults in the US have reported symptoms of anxiety or depressive disorders [39]. Self-isolation can lead to anxiety, depression, public anger, and post-traumatic stress disorder (PTSD). When this stress is combined with other destabilizing factors, such as economic problems and the fear of getting infected, the result is a very strong psychological impact on the global population. Moreover, the increased stress in healthcare workers and other essential workers, unemployment consequences, and financial difficulties are additional factors that can lead to several psychological problems in selected categories [40, 41]. This phenomenon has already been extensively verified after previous outbreaks such as the SARS in 2002 [42]. On the other hand, evidence suggests that psychological sequelae and/or a long-term functional impairment may be due to the disease itself [43, 44]. Nevertheless, it is currently difficult to establish how much of these mental health consequences is secondary to the disease (e.g., through neuroinflammatory processes) or not. Since the single mechanisms can cross each other, the phenomenon has probably a multifactorial genesis. Clinical and epidemiological research will clear up many doubts on this hot topic.

Despite these limitations, this section presents an overview of the psychological issues in those who have had the disease. These clinical manifestations are referred to as long-COVID problems. For similar issues affecting the general population, the reader can refer to other sources [39].

Another premise concerns the terminology used. Throughout the text, the term "Psychiatric" is used to describe disorders, symptoms, and signs listed within the category "Chapter 06, Mental, Behavioral and Neurodevelopmental Disorders" from the 11th Revision of the International Classification of Diseases and Related Health Problems (ICD-11) of the World Health Organization (WHO). It includes symptoms such as mood disorders, anxiety and fear-related disorders, and disorders specifically associated with stress [45]. On the contrary, the term "Neuropsychiatric" should more properly be used for indicating psychiatric disorders, symptoms, and signs that are the result of brain damage or disease. Therefore, neuropsychiatric consequences must necessarily include damage to the nervous tissue produced directly by the viral action, or triggered and sustained by a more or less extensive neuroinflammation processes. In the current uncertainty about the mechanisms of neurotoxicity, here we prefer to focus the reader's attention on the clinical aspects, rather than investigating the pathogenesis of the phenomenon. In other chapters of the book, more in-depth details are offered.

4.4.2 From Acute to Chronic Psychiatric Problems

During the acute or short-term post-illness phases of the COVID-19, several studies focused on the occurrence of psychiatric problems. Crunfli et al. [46] reported that affective disorders and anxiety involved 20% and 28% of the patients, respectively. Nevertheless, as Xie et al. [47] stated, most investigations on mental health problems associated with acute COVID-19 have serious limitations, such as the small sample size, and the lack of an exhaustive assessed of psychiatric symptoms through psychiatric interviews. They performed a meta-analysis of studies assessing psychiatric symptoms and found that, in the acute stage, psychiatric problems were mainly acute stress reactions, such as somatization, phobia, and appetite and sleep disorders. Although these symptoms were of medium-to-severe severity, they can be easily manageable if properly treated. This finding imposes a careful psychiatric assessment which must be performed by using adequate tools and administered by specialized personnel [47].

Notably, in the course of illness, a new diagnosis of psychiatric pathology was made in many young people [48]. The underlying causes of this finding are difficult to establish and only hypotheses can be proposed. For instance, since encephalitis alone can lead to an increased risk of a variety of long-term sequelae, such as bipolar disorders, psychotic disorders, anxiety disorders, cognitive problems, and dementia [49], it is reasonable to expect a high incidence of psychiatric pathologies in those who have experienced diffuse inflammatory processes including neuroinflammation. However, encephalitis is not a common finding among the manifestations of neuro-COVID.

Regardless of the cause and type of psychiatric sequelae, it seems to be difficult to establish the extent of chronic neuropsychiatric sequelae. Pending the results of long-term follow-up investigations, it is possible to speculate by using data from studies on previous endemics and, above all, on the effects produced on mental health in ICU survivors. After the ICU discharge, a complex neuropsychiatric picture can develop. This syndrome, which is indicated as post-intensive care syndrome (PICS), affects the physical, cognitive, and psychological health status [50]. Symptoms of PICS are manifold and can include a different combination of neuromuscular disorders, such as generalized weakness (classified as critical illness myopathy, neuropathy, and neuromyopathy), with cognitive and psychological problems, such as memory disturbances, poor concentration ("brain fog"), depression, and anxiety. Of note, PTSD can be also encompassed among the PICS disorders [51]. About the extent of the problem, it has been estimated that the PICS can affect up to 60% of post-ICU patients [50]. Among the long-COVID issues, the PICS phenomenon must be very carefully evaluated due to both the high incidence and clinical consequences. Interestingly, up to 20% of COVID-19 patients require hospitalization [52] and, of those, up to one-quarter need ICU admission [53]. Furthermore, from other sources, it emerges that the ICU admission ranges from 5% of all of those testing positive in China [54] to 12% in Italy [55]. Thus, we can aspect an incredible number of long-COVID individuals with PICS, worldwide. Moreover, in the context of COVID-19, dedicated programs aimed at preventing the onset of PICS, such as open-ICU, early rehabilitation, light sedation, and prevention of delirium, can hardly be implemented. The severity of the respiratory failure, the high number of patients admitted, and the need to impede the presence of relatives in the ward represent great obstacles. Since the PICS can last many years, the effects on the QoL in post-COVID subjects and the socioeconomic impact can be devastating [56].

In COVID survivors, a special issue concerns PTSD. It is an acute, disabling mental disorder that develops after exposure to a life-threatening traumatic event [57]. Clinically, the symptoms usually appear within 3 months of the trauma although sometimes the state of stress can occur later. Symptoms can be classified into four well-defined categories:

- *Intrusive memories.* People with PTSD have sudden memories that manifest themselves vividly and are accompanied by painful emotions and the "reliving" of the drama. Sometimes, the experience is so strong that it seems to the individual involved that the traumatic event is repeating itself.
- *Avoidance.* The person tries to avoid contact with anyone and anything that brings him back to the trauma. Initially, the person experiences an emotional state of disinterest and detachment, reducing his capacity for emotional interaction and being able to conduct only simple and routine activities. The lack of emotional processing causes an accumulation of anxiety and tension that can become chronic, leading to real depressive states. At the same time, guilt frequently arises.
- *Alterations in cognition and mood.* There is often an inability to remember important aspects of the traumatic event. Moreover, negative thoughts and feelings leading to ongoing and distorted beliefs about oneself or others can manifest. Again, distorted thoughts about the cause or consequences of the event that lead to wrongly blaming oneself or others, continued fear, horror, anger, or

shame, less interest in previously enjoyed activities as well as feeling detached or estranged from others may be present.

- *Alterations in arousal and reactivity*. People behave as if they are constantly threatened by trauma. They react violently and suddenly, cannot concentrate, have memory problems and constantly feel in danger. Sometimes, to relieve their pain, people turn to alcohol or drug use. A person with PTSD can also lose control over their life and, therefore, can be at risk for suicidal behavior.

Critical care admission is a well-recognized cause of this syndrome. Recently, it was demonstrated that, in the setting of ICU, about 20% of discharged patients will develop PTSD [58]. The diagnosis of post-ICU PTSD is of fundamental importance, as if not properly treated, it can significantly worsen the QoL. Notably, several pharmacological and non-pharmacological approaches can be very helpful in the treatment of PTSD [59]. About the incidence of PTSD in COVID-19, Bo et al. [60] showed that the syndrome can develop in most hospitalized patients (96%). Nevertheless, the in-hospital assessment cannot allow an accurate estimate of the phenomenon as the patient is still subjected to the acute stress of hospitalization. In another study conducted in hospitalized, treated and discharged patients, the prevalence rate of PTSD was 20.3% [61]. Tarsitani et al. [62] performed a precise analysis and assessed the prevalence of PTSD at 3-month follow-up after hospital discharge through the PTSD Checklist for DSM-5 (PCL-5) [63]. Although they found a prevalence of 10%, in another 8.6% of the sample a diagnosis of subthreshold PTSD was obtained. This data is of great importance as the latter disorder can lead to significant levels of distress and impairment.

About risk factors for PTSD development following COVID-19, there are a previous psychiatric diagnosis and obesity. Moreover, the male gender seems to be a protective factor [61]. Interestingly, several investigations demonstrated that young to middle-aged women are more prone to long-COVID [64]. This phenomenon can have several explanations. According to the "pregnancy compensation hypothesis," for example, women of reproductive age have more reactive immune responses to pathogen as their immune systems have evolved to support the heightened need for protection during pregnancy [65]. Furthermore, autoimmune processes are more evident in the female gender [66].

Another risk factor is probably the degree of the disease and mostly the dyspnea during hospitalization [67]. A recent cross-sectional online survey evaluated the psychological impacts on the quarantine/isolation experience of participants suspected or confirmed to have COVID-19, their PTSD status, and several correlate with developing PTSD [68]. The authors found lower rates of PTSD symptoms in participants practicing religion (Buddhist) than in participants having no religion (OR: 0.30; 95% CI: 0.13–0.68; $p = 0.005$). Moreover, compared to those voluntarily quarantined/isolated, subjects forced to be quarantined/isolated had an increased risk of developing PTSD symptoms. Further, having a positive diagnosis of the infection was a predictive factor of stress during pandemics. This latter finding confirmed that stress symptoms are more severe in COVID-19 survivors compared to healthy controls [69]. Interestingly, it seems that there are no differences between healthcare workers and non-healthcare workers in PTSD scores [68], but it is not possible to generalize as the risk of psychological distress appears to be particularly high in some categories such as those involved in the care of critically ill patients [70].

Taken together, these findings suggest that careful attention must be paid to post-COVID patients. The assessment of the psychiatric problems, indeed, must be conducted through dedicated tools and respecting the appropriate timelines. For example, it was reported that following SARS, although the prevalence of PTSD was about 5% at the 3-month follow-up, this percentage increased to over 25% after 30 months from the discharge [71]. Thus, since psychiatric symptoms manifested during the acute phase of the disease may persist for a long time after discharge, regular monitoring of psychiatric symptoms, as well as psychosocial support and/or ad hoc psychiatric treatment may be required [47].

4.5 Potential Long-Term Cognitive Issues

Several cognitive problems such as "brain fog" and complex dysexecutive symptoms have been described as complications of COVID-19. The "brain fog" is not a medical condition as the term is generically used to refer to a cognitive dysfunction because of other clinical conditions. It involves memory problems, lack of mental clarity, poor concentration, and inability to focus. Dysexecutive symptoms are a set of symptoms that include cognitive, behavioral, and emotional problems. They manifest as a dysfunction in executive functions, such as planning, thinking, and behavioral control. In the context of post-COVID, neurocognitive issues are of paramount importance. For example, in their meta-analysis Roger et al. [72] found that confusion and agitation affected, respectively, 65% and 69% of ICU-patients; moreover, one-third of the patients manifested dysexecutive syndromes at discharge. This alteration in mental status can reflect encephalopathy/encephalitis mechanism and primary psychiatric diagnoses, especially in young patients [48]. Furthermore, an impaired memory was found in 28% of the patients [46].

Although the incidence and features of the long-term cognitive effects should be evaluated through dedicated follow-up studies, the literature can suggest several arguments of discussion on the underlying mechanisms. Hypoperfusion in the frontotemporal region of the brain and structural brain abnormalities involving the thalamic and temporal regions described in ICU COVID-19 patients can play an important role [73].

Moreover, the increasing knowledge of the pathophysiology of COVID-19 has raised some concerns about the link between the infection and neurodegenerative diseases such as dementia, multiple sclerosis, and Parkinson's disease (PD). Although it is not yet clear if the SARS-CoV-2 virus could cause or accelerate their occurrence, many potential pathological mechanisms could be involved. Probably, this coronavirus could have a role in promoting a chronic immune and inflammatory response in the brain, leading to neurodegenerative changes even after months or years [74]. Additionally, Gordon et al. [75] showed the effects of SARS-CoV-2 on aging hallmarks. In particular, several SARS-CoV-2 proteins including the spike can interfere with a variety of aging-related pathways such as ubiquitin ligases, vesicle trafficking systems, lipid modifications pathways, and RNA processing and mitochondrial activities. Thus, damages are produced by the endoplasmic reticulum stress, mitochondrial dysfunction, and loss of proteostasis with autophagy deficiency.

On the other hand, the severity of disease, the ICU stay, and therapies (e.g., glucocorticoids) can unmask an underlying neurodegenerative process. In this context, the emergence of cognitive or non-cognitive symptoms (e.g., neurological manifestations) following the acute phase of COVID-19 can help anticipate a diagnosis. For example, several clinical manifestations such as chronic pain [76], fatigue, and sleep disorders following COVID-19 may represent non-motor symptoms of PD. Again, in this neurodegenerative disease, loss of olfaction is considered an early manifestation [77]. As suggested by Lippi et al. [78] SARS-CoV-2 can stay at a crossroad between aging and neurodegeneration. In addition to the neuroinflammation and altered immunity processes, as well as to the direct aging-promoting role of the SARS-CoV-2, other factors can intersect in the possible pathogenetic cascade. In fact, during the acute or post-illness phases of the COVID-19 neurocognitive symptoms might be exacerbated due to social and environmental effects.

Notably, long-term neurocognitive issues are not inherent the elderly and/or those who have suffered from particularly severe forms of the disease. It can also regard young and middle-aged adults who were never hospitalized during acute COVID-19. Furthermore, data from the Long-term Impact of Infection with Novel Coronavirus (LIINC) study in San Francisco, US, underline that in this population cognitive symptoms may be common last up to several months after recovering from the acute phase of COVID-19 [18]. Since these cognitive problems can be difficult to intercept by the classic 30-point Mini Mental State Exam (MMSE), a careful assessment requires a combination of tools.

Considering the huge impact on health-associated functioning and QoL, the long-COVID issue must be carefully addressed [78]. About symptoms of neuro-COVID, in a recent systematic review, Nasserie et al. [79] found that median proportion of individuals who experienced at least 1 persistent symptom was 73%. Of these, fatigue with a median frequency of 40%; and sleep disorders/insomnia 30%. Consequently, management of long haulers from neuro-COVID requires a multiprofessional approach that involves neurologists, pain therapists, nutritionists, neuroradiologists, physical therapists, otolaryngologists, and others. Follow-ups must be carefully scheduled in those who have suffered from the more severe forms of the disease and in individuals who have had mild or moderate COVID-19 acute manifestations. Since all aspects of QoL need to be evaluated, it is worth referring to a battery of tools. Therapy should focus on the type of disorder. For example, chronic pain requires multimodal treatment by pain therapists [80]; smell disorders are managed through rehabilitation programs, and psychological and neurological problems are addressed by specialists. Individuals suspected of PICS/PTSD need early rehabilitation and a mental assessment at the acute and post-acute phase. Nutritional evaluation also plays an important role. In particular, vitamins, polyphenols [81], ω-3 fatty acids, minerals, and low glycemic index foods have an inhibitory action against oxidative stress and neuroinflammation and can positively influence cognitive function [82].

Practical Suggestions for Addressing Neurological, Psychological, and Cognitive Manifestations of Long-COVID

- Multiprofessional approach (nurses, neurologists, pain therapists, nutritionists, neuroradiologists, physical therapists, occupational therapists, otolaryngologists, and others).
- Neuroimaging, if appropriate.
- Laboratory tests, if appropriate.
- Appropriate and timely individualized therapy (e.g., anticoagulation for neurological signs and symptoms suggestive of post-COVID stroke).
- Long-term follow-up (1–2 years, or more).
- Careful psychological/neurocognitive assessment through a combination of tools:
  - *Short Form Health Survey 36 (SF-36)*: it evaluates physical functioning, social functioning, limitations due to physical problems, limitations due to emotional problems, mental health, energy/vitality, pain, and perception of general health (6 items). It is useful for assessing the health changes compared to the previous year.
  - *Barthel Index*: it measures improvements in individuals with chronic disability who underwent rehabilitation programs (e.g., in post-ICU individuals).
  - *Psychological General Well-Being Index (PGWBI)*: it evaluates the subjective well-being or suffering by assessing anxiety, depression, positive well-being, self-control, general health, and vitality.
  - *EuroQoL*: it evaluates HRQoL regardless of the specific disease.
  - *Pittsburgh Sleep Quality Index (PSQI)*: it assesses the sleep quality.
  - *Mini Mental State Exam (MMSE)*: it investigates on the neurocognitive and functional state by exploring domains of brain function (e.g., orientation, memory, attention and calculation, ability to recall acquisitions, language).
  - *Brief Pain Inventory (BPI)*: it assesses the severity of pain and its impact on functioning.
  - *Post-Traumatic Stress Syndrome 14 items (PTSS-14):* it is a screening tool for PTSD.
  - *Symptom Checklist-90-Revised (SCL-90-R):* it is a widely used self-report scale to assess a broad range of psychological problems and symptoms of psychopathology.
  - *Hospital Anxiety and Depression Scale (HADS):* it evaluates depression and anxiety.
  - *Mini Nutritional Assessment (MNA)*: it assesses nutritional status.
- Rehabilitation programs.
- Nutritional strategies.

4.6 Conclusions

The emerging condition of persistent symptomatology following the acute phase of COVID-19 has become of primary importance for health care systems. The millions of people involved in the infection and the evidence that even the mildest forms of the disease could be followed by a long-lasting and debilitating symptomatology, require an early and comprehensive approach to this condition. The public health implications could be considerable and the crashing wave of neurological and/or neuropsychiatric sequelae of COVID can have the effect of a tsunami. A starting point for addressing the phenomenon is to characterize the symptoms and the various clinical expressions of the long-term health impairment. Neurological symptoms such as fatigue and muscle weakness, psychological conditions, including sleep disorders, anxiety, and depression, as well as neurocognitive problems can persist for months and can range from mild issues to serious and debilitating disorders. Data on the incidence of single symptoms and the duration of each clinical picture after the acute phase vary greatly according to the type of study carried out, the timing, and the setting investigated. Therefore, it is mandatory to establish diagnostic criteria and methodology of study that can be universally accepted. For this purpose, the role of scientific societies is of fundamental importance.

References

1. National Institute for Health and Care Excellence (NICE). (2020). COVID-19 rapid guideline: managing the long-term effects of COVID-19. Published: 18 December 2020 wwwniceorguk/guidance/ng188, last accessed: May 29, 2021.
2. Leung TYM, Chan AYL, Chan EW, et al. Short- and potential long-term adverse health outcomes of COVID-19: a rapid review. Emerg Microbes Infect. 2020;9(1):2190–9. https://doi.org/10.1080/22221751.2020.1825914.
3. Alwan NA, Johnson L. Defining long COVID: going back to the start. Med (N Y). 2021;2(5):501–4. https://doi.org/10.1016/j.medj.2021.03.003.
4. Fernández-de-las-Peñas C, Palacios-Ceña D, Gómez-Mayordomo V, et al. Defining post-COVID symptoms (post-acute COVID, long COVID, persistent post-COVID): an integrative classification. J Environ Res Public Health. 2021;18(5):2621. https://doi.org/10.3390/ijerph18052621.
5. Nalbandian A, Sehgal K, Gupta A, et al. Post-acute COVID-19 syndrome. Nat Med. 2021;27(4):601–15. https://doi.org/10.1038/s41591-021-01283-z.
6. Mahase E. Long COVID could be four different syndromes, review suggests. BMJ. 2020;2020(371):m3981.
7. Mahase E. COVID-19: what do we know about "long COVID"? BMJ. 2020;370:m2815.
8. Nabavi N. Long covid: how to define it and how to manage it. BMJ. 2020;370:m3489.
9. Greenhalgh T, Knight M, A'Court C, et al. Management of post-acute covid-19 in primary care. BMJ. 2020;370:m3026.
10. Nehme M, Braillard O, Alcoba G, et al. COVID19 symptoms: longitudinal evolution and persistence in outpatient settings. Ann Intern Med. 2021;174(5):723–5. https://doi.org/10.7326/M20-5926.
11. Tenforde MV, Kim SS, Lindsell CJ, et al. Symptom duration and risk factors for delayed return to usual health among outpatients with COVID-19 in a multistate health care systems network—

United States, March–June 2020. MMWR Morb Mortal Wkly Rep. 2020;69(30):993–8. https://doi.org/10.15585/mmwr.mm6930e1.
12. Carfì A, Bernabei R, Landi F, et al. Persistent symptoms in patients after acute COVID-19. JAMA. 2020;324(6):603–5. https://doi.org/10.1001/jama.2020.12603.
13. Office for National Statistics (2020). Prevalence of long COVID symptoms and COVID-19 complications https://www.ons.gov.uk/peoplepopulationandcommunity/healthandsocialcare/healthandlifeexpectancies/datasets/prevalenceoflongcovidsymptomsandcovid19complications. last accessed May 26, 2021.
14. Assaf G, Davis H, McCorkell L, et al (2020) What does COVID-19 recovery actually look like? An analysis of the prolonged COVID-19 symptoms. Survey by patient-led research team. https://patientresearchcovid19.com, last accessed June 20,2021.
15. Goërtz YMJ, Van Herck M, Delbressine JM, et al. Persistent symptoms 3 months after a SARS-CoV-2 infection: the post-COVID-19 syndrome? ERJ Open Res. 2020;6:00542–2020. https://doi.org/10.1183/23120541.00542-2020.
16. Davis AE, Assaf GF, Mc Corkell L, et al. Characterizing long COVID in an international cohort: 7 months of symptoms and their impact. medRxiv. preprint. 2021; https://doi.org/10.1101/2020.12.24.20248802.
17. Cirulli E, Barrett KMS, Riffle S, et al. Long-term COVID-19 symptoms in a large unselected population. medRxiv. 2020; https://doi.org/10.1101/2020.10.07.20208702.
18. Hellmuth J, Barnett TA, Asken BM, et al. Persistent COVID-19-associated neurocognitive symptoms in non-hospitalized patients. J Neurovirol. 2021;27(1):191–5. https://doi.org/10.1007/s13365-021-00954-4.
19. Chopra V, Flanders SA, O'Malley M, et al. Sixty-day outcomes among patients hospitalized with COVID-19. Ann Intern Med. 2020;174(4):576–8. https://doi.org/10.7326/m20-5661.
20. Logue JK, Franko NM, McCulloch DJ, et al. Sequelae in adults at 6 months after COVID-19 infection. JAMA Netw Open. 2021;4(2):e210830. https://doi.org/10.1001/jamanetworkopen.2021.0830.
21. Wang F, Kream RM, Stefano GB. Long-term respiratory and neurological sequelae of COVID-19. Med Sci Monit. 2020;26:e928996. https://doi.org/10.12659/MSM.928996.
22. Wijeratne T, Crewther S. Post-COVID 19 neurological syndrome (PCNS); a novel syndrome with challenges for the global neurology community. J Neurol Sci. 2020;419:117179. https://doi.org/10.1016/j.jns.2020.117179.
23. Baig AM. Deleterious outcomes in long-hauler COVID-19: the effects of SARS-CoV-2 on the CNS in chronic COVID syndrome. ACS Chem Neurosci. 2020;11(24):4017–20. https://doi.org/10.1021/acschemneuro.0c00725.
24. Doykov I, Hällqvist J, Gilmour KC, et al. 'The long tail of Covid-19'—the detection of a prolonged inflammatory response after a SARS-CoV-2 infection in asymptomatic and mildly affected patients. F1000Res. 2020;9:1349. https://doi.org/10.12688/f1000research.27287.2.
25. Sun B, Tang N, Peluso MJ, et al. Characterization and biomarker analyses of post-COVID-19 complications and neurological manifestations. Cell. 2021;10(2):386. https://doi.org/10.3390/cells10020386.
26. Bossù P, Toppi E, Sterbini V, et al. Implication of aging related chronic Neuroinflammation on COVID-19 pandemic. J Pers Med. 2020;10:102. https://doi.org/10.3390/jpm10030102.
27. Rudroff T, Fietsam AC, Deters JR, Bryant AD, Kamholz J. Post-COVID-19 fatigue: potential contributing factors. Brain Sci. 2020;10(12):1012. https://doi.org/10.3390/brainsci10121012.
28. Kamal M, Omirah MA, Hussein A, et al. Assessment and characterisation of post-COVID-19 manifestations. Int J Clin Pract. 2021;75:e13746. https://doi.org/10.1111/ijcp.13746.
29. Huang C, Huang L, Wang Y, et al. 6-month consequences of COVID-19 in patients discharged from hospital: a cohort study. Lancet. 2021;397(10270):220–32. https://doi.org/10.1016/S0140-6736(20)32656-8.
30. Vittori A, Lerman J, Cascella M, et al. COVID-19 pandemic acute respiratory distress syndrome survivors: pain after the storm? Anesth Analg. 2020;131(1):117–9. https://doi.org/10.1213/ANE.0000000000004914.

31. Clauw DJ, Hauser W, Cohen SP, et al. Considering the potential for an increase in chronic pain after the COVID-19 pandemic. Pain. 2020;161(8):1694–7. https://doi.org/10.1097/j.pain.0000000000001950.
32. Kemp HI, Corner E, Colvin LA. Chronic pain after COVID-19: implications for rehabilitation. BJA. 2020;125(4):436e449. https://doi.org/10.1016/j.bja.2020.05.021.
33. Belvis R. Headaches during COVID-19: my clinical case and review of the literature. Headache. 2020;60(7):1422–6. https://doi.org/10.1111/head.13841.
34. Uygun O, Ertaş M, Ekizoğlu E, et al. Headache characteristics in COVID-19 pandemic—a survey study. J Headache Pain. 2020;21:121. https://doi.org/10.1186/s10194-020-01188-1.
35. Sheehy LM. Considerations for Postacute rehabilitation for survivors of COVID-19. JMIR Public Health Surveill. 2020;6(2):e19462. https://doi.org/10.2196/19462.
36. Raahimi MM, Kane A, Moore CEG, et al. Late onset of Guillain-Barré syndrome following SARS-CoV-2 infection: part of 'long COVID-19 syndrome'? BMJ Case Rep. 2021;14:e240178. https://doi.org/10.1136/bcr-2020-240178.
37. Nalleballe K, Reddy Onteddu S, Sharma R, Dandu V, et al. Spectrum of neuropsychiatric manifestations in COVID-19. Brain Behav Immun. 2020;88:71–4. https://doi.org/10.1016/j.bbi.2020.06.020.
38. Kincaid KJ, Kung JC, Senetar AJ, et al. Post-COVID seizure: a new feature of "long-COVID". eNeurological Sci. 2021;23:100340. https://doi.org/10.1016/j.ensci.2021.100340.
39. Kearney A, Hamel L, Brodie M. Mental Health Impact of the COVID-19 Pandemic: an update. KFF analysis. Available at: https://www.kff.org/coronavirus-covid-19/poll-finding/mental-health-impact-of-the-covid-19-pandemic/. Last accessed: May 12, 2021.
40. Greenberg N, Docherty M, Gnanapragasam S, Wessely S. Managing mental health challenges faced by healthcare workers during covid-19 pandemic. BMJ. 2020;368:m1211. https://doi.org/10.1136/bmj.m1211.
41. Chaves C, Castellanos T, Abrams M, Vazquez C. The impact of economic recessions on depression and individual and social well-being: the case of Spain (2006–2013). Soc Psychiatry Psychiatr Epidemiol. 2018;53:977–86.
42. Siu JY. The SARS-associated stigma of SARS victims in the post-SARS era of Hong Kong. Qual Health Res. 2008;18:729–38.
43. Mirfazeli FS, Sarabi-Jamab A, Jahanbakhshi A, et al. Neuropsychiatric manifestations of COVID-19 can be clustered in three distinct symptom categories. Sci Rep. 2020;10(1):20957. https://doi.org/10.1038/s41598-020-78050-6.
44. Kumar S, Veldhuis A, Malhotra T. Neuropsychiatric and cognitive sequelae of COVID-19. Front Psychol. 2021;12:577529. https://doi.org/10.3389/fpsyg.2021.577529.
45. WHO. (2018). The ICD-11 classification of mental and behavioural disorders: clinical descriptions and diagnostic guidelines. Available at: https://icdwhoint/en. Last accessed June 12, 2021.
46. Crunfli F, Carregari VC, Veras FP, et al. SARS-CoV-2 infects brain astrocytes of COVID-19 patients and impairs neuronal viability. medRxiv [preprint]. 2020; https://doi.org/10.1101/2020.10.09.20207464.
47. Xie Q, Liu XB, Xu YM, et al. Understanding the psychiatric symptoms of COVID-19: a meta-analysis of studies assessing psychiatric symptoms in Chinese patients with and survivors of COVID-19 and SARS by using the symptom Checklist-90-revised. Transl Psychiatry. 2021;11:290. https://doi.org/10.1038/s41398-021-01416-5.
48. Varatharaj A, Thomas N, Ellul M, et al. UK-wide surveillance of neurological and neuropsychiatric complications of COVID-19: the first 153 patients. SSRN [Preprint]; 2020. https://doi.org/10.2139/ssrn.3601761.
49. Ballard C, Orrell M, YongZhong S. Impact of antipsychotic review and nonpharmacological intervention on antipsychotic use, neuropsychiatric symptoms, and mortality in people with dementia living in nursing homes: a factorial cluster-randomized controlled trial by the Well-being and health for people with dementia (WHELD) program. Am J Psychiatry. 2016;173:252–62.
50. Rawal G, Yadav S, Kumar R. Post-intensive care syndrome: an overview. J Transl Int Med. 2017;5(2):90–2.

51. Righy C, Rosa RG, da Silva RTA, et al. Prevalence of post-traumatic stress disorder symptoms in adult critical care survivors: a systematic review and meta-analysis. Crit Care. 2019;23(1):213. https://doi.org/10.1186/s13054-019-2489-3.
52. Nanjayya V. Report of the WHO-China joint Mission on coronavirus disease 2019 (COVID-19). WHO-China Jt Mission Coronavirus Dis 2019. 2020;2019:16–24. Available at: https://wwwwhoint/docs/default-source/coronaviruse/who-china-joint-mission-on-covid-19-final-reportpdf. Last accessed: May 29, 2021
53. UpToDate. Coronavirus Disease 2019 (COVID-19): Critical Care and Airway Management Issues. Available at: https://www.uptodate.com/contents/coronavirus-disease-2019-covid-19-critical-care-and-airway-management-issues Last accessed: May 29, 2021.
54. Wu Y, Xu X, Chen Z, Duan J, Hashimoto K, Yang L, et al. Nervous system involvement after infection with COVID-19 and other coronaviruses. Brain Behav Immun. 2020;87:18–22. https://doi.org/10.1016/j.bbi.2020.03.031.
55. Grasselli G, Zangrillo A, Zanella A, et al. Baseline characteristics and outcomes of 1591 patients infected with SARS-CoV-2 admitted to ICUs of the Lombardy region, Italy. J Am Med Assoc. 2020;323(16):1574–81.
56. Kamdar BB, Suri R, Suchyta MR, et al. Return to work after critical illness: a systematic review and meta-analysis. Thorax. 2020;75(1):17–27.
57. American Psychiatric Association. American Psychiatric Association: diagnostic and statistical manual of mental disorders. 5th ed; 2013.
58. Righy C, Rosa RG, Da Silva RTA, et al. Prevalence of post-traumatic stress disorder symptoms in adult critical care survivors: a systematic review and meta-analysis. Crit Care. 2019;23(1):1–13.
59. Bryant RA. Post-traumatic stress disorder: a state-of-the-art review of evidence and challenges. World Psychiatry. 2019;18(3):259–69.
60. Bo HX, Li W, Yang Y, et al. Posttraumatic stress symptoms and attitude toward crisis mental health services among clinically stable patients with COVID-19 in China. Psychol Med. 2020;51(6):1052–3. https://doi.org/10.1017/S0033291720000999.
61. Chang MC, Park D. Incidence of post-traumatic stress disorder after coronavirus disease. Healthcare (Basel). 2020;8(4):373. https://doi.org/10.3390/healthcare8040373.
62. Tarsitani L, Vassalini P, Koukopoulos A, et al. Post-traumatic stress disorder among COVID-19 survivors at 3-month follow-up after hospital discharge. J Gen Intern Med. 2021;29:1–6. https://doi.org/10.1007/s11606-021-06731-7.
63. Weathers FW, Litz BT, Keane TM, et al. The PTSD checklist for DSM-5 (PCL-5). National Center for PTSD. Published online 2013; 2013. https://doi.org/10.1037/t02622-000.
64. Torjesen I. Covid-19: middle aged women face greater risk of debilitating long term symptoms. BMJ. 2021;372:n829. https://doi.org/10.1136/bmj.n829.
65. Natri H, Garcia AR, Buetow KH, Trumble BC, Wilson MA. The pregnancy pickle: evolved immune compensation due to pregnancy underlies sex differences in human diseases. Trends Genet. 2019;35(7):478–88. https://doi.org/10.1016/j.tig.2019.04.008.
66. Khamsi R. Rogue antibodies could be driving severe COVID-19. Nature. 2021;590(7844):29–31. https://doi.org/10.1038/d41586-021-00149-1.
67. Einvik G, Dammen T, Ghanima W, Heir T, Stavem K. Prevalence and risk factors for post-traumatic stress in hospitalized and non-hospitalized COVID-19 patients. Int J Environ Res Public Health. 2021;18(4):2079.
68. Tmgh-Global Covid-Collaborative. Psychological impacts and post-traumatic stress disorder among people under COVID-19 quarantine and isolation: a global survey. Int J Environ Res Public Health. 2021;18(11):5719. https://doi.org/10.3390/ijerph18115719.
69. Yuan Y, Liu ZH, Zhao YJ, et al. Prevalence of post-traumatic stress symptoms and its associations with quality of life, demographic and clinical characteristics in COVID-19 survivors during the post-COVID-19 era. Front Psych. 2021;12:665507. https://doi.org/10.3389/fpsyt.2021.665507.
70. Vittori A, Marchetti G, Pedone R, et al. COVID-19 pandemic mental health risks among anesthesiologists: it is not only burnout. Braz J Anesthesiol. 2021;71(2):201–3. https://doi.org/10.1016/j.bjane.2021.01.002.

71. Wu P, Fang Y, Guan Z, et al. The psychological impact of the SARS epidemic on hospital employees in China: exposure, risk perception, and altruistic acceptance of risk. Can J Psychiatr. 2009;54(5):302–11.
72. Rogers JP, Chesney E, Oliver D, Pollak TA, McGuire P, Fusar-Poli P, et al. Psychiatric and neuropsychiatric presentations associated with severe coronavirus infections: a systematic review and meta-analysis with comparison to the COVID-19 pandemic. Lancet Psychiatry. 2020;7:611–27. https://doi.org/10.1016/S2215-0366(20)30203-0.
73. Helms J, Kremer S, Merdji H, Clere-Jehl R, Schenck M, Kummerlen C, et al. Neurologic features in severe SARS-CoV-2 infection. N Engl J Med. 2020;382:2268–70.
74. Calderòn-Garciduenas L, Torres-Jardòn R, Franco-Lira M, et al. Environmental nanoparticles, SARS-CoV-2 brain involvement, and potential acceleration of Alzheimer's and Parkinson's diseases in young urbanites exposed to air pollution. J Alzheimers Dis. 2020;78:479–503. https://doi.org/10.3233/JAD-200891.
75. Gordon DE, Jang GM, Bouhaddou M, et al. A SARS-CoV-2-human protein-protein interaction map reveals drug targets and potential drug-repurposing. Biorxiv. 2020; 2020.03.22.002386v1. [preprint]
76. Cuomo A, Crispo A, Truini A, et al. Toward more focused multimodal and multidisciplinary approaches for pain management in Parkinson's disease. J Pain Res. 2019;12:2201–9. https://doi.org/10.2147/JPR.S209616.
77. Doty RL. Olfaction in Parkinson's disease and related disorders. Neurobiol Dis. 2012;46:527–52.
78. Lippi A, Domingues R, Setz C, Outeiro TF, Krisko A. SARS-CoV-2: at the crossroad between aging and neurodegeneration. Mov Disord. 2020;35(5):716–20. https://doi.org/10.1002/mds.28084.
78. Crispo A, Bimonte S, Porciello G, et al. Strategies to evaluate outcomes in long-COVID-19 and post-COVID survivors. Infect Agent Cancer. 2021;16(1):62. https://doi.org/10.1186/s13027-021-00401-3.
79. Nasserie T, Hittle M, Goodman SN. Assessment of the frequency and variety of persistent symptoms among patients with COVID-19: a systematic review. JAMA Netw Open. 2021;4(5):e2111417. https://doi.org/10.1001/jamanetworkopen.2021.11417.
80. Cuomo A, Bimonte S, Forte CA, Botti G, Cascella M. Multimodal approaches and tailored therapies for pain management: the trolley analgesic model. J Pain Res. 2019;12:711–4. https://doi.org/10.2147/JPR.S178910.
81. Cascella M, Bimonte S, Barbieri A, et al. Dissecting the potential roles of Nigella sativa and its constituent Thymoquinone on the prevention and on the progression of Alzheimer's disease. Front Aging Neurosci. 2018;10:16. https://doi.org/10.3389/fnagi.2018.00016.
82. Miquel S, Champ C, Day J, et al. Poor cognitive ageing: vulnerabilities, mechanisms and the impact of nutritional interventions. Ageing Res Rev. 2018;2:40–55. https://doi.org/10.1016/j.arr.2017.12.004.

MIX
Papier aus verantwortungsvollen Quellen
Paper from responsible sources
FSC® C105338

If you have any concerns about our products,
you can contact us on
ProductSafety@springernature.com

In case Publisher is established outside the EU,
the EU authorized representative is:
Springer Nature Customer Service Center GmbH
Europaplatz 3, 69115 Heidelberg, Germany

Printed by Libri Plureos GmbH
in Hamburg, Germany